REVIVING
PRIMARY
CARE

A US-UK COMPARISON

JOHN FRY

WHO Consultant in Primary Care, and former Member
of Council, Royal College of General Practitioners, UK

DONALD LIGHT

Professor of Comparative Health Care Systems, University
of Medicine and Dentistry of New Jersey, Camden, USA

JONATHAN RODNICK

Professor and Chair, Department of Family and
Community Medicine, University of California,
San Francisco, USA

PETER ORTON

Immediate Past-President of the General Practice Section,
The Royal Society of Medicine, and General Practitioner,
Hatfield Heath, Essex, UK

FOREWORD BY
ROBERT S LAWRENCE

Director, Health Sciences, Rockefeller Foundation, USA

RADCLIFFE MEDICAL PRESS
OXFORD AND NEW YORK

© 1995 John Fry, Donald Light, Jonathan Rodnick, Peter Orton

Radcliffe Medical Press Ltd
18 Marcham Road, Abingdon, Oxon, OX14 1AA, UK

Radcliffe Medical Press, Inc.
141 Fifth Avenue, New York, NY 10010, USA

British Library Cataloguing in Publication Data

A catalogue record for this book is available from the British Library.

ISBN 1 85775 001 2

Library of Congress Cataloging-in-Publication Data is available.

Typeset by Acorn Bookwork, Salisbury, Wiltshire

Dedicated to the memory of John Fry, a generous spirit and a master of general practice who, through careful observations of his practice and other practices around the world, moved primary care forward in an era of specialization.

Contents

Contents

Authors' Biographies

John Fry was Britain's most distinguished general practitioner and known throughout the world for his writings about comparative primary care.

Donald Light is an American sociologist internationally known for his work on comparative health care systems. He is a professor at the University of Medicine and Dentistry of New Jersey, and an adjunct senior fellow at the Leonard Davis Institute of Health Economics.

Jonathan Rodnick is a leading practitioner and professor at the University of California, San Francisco, School of Medicine, where he chairs the Department of Family and Community Medicine.

Peter Orton is Immediate Past-President of the General Practice Section, The Royal Society of Medicine, and a general practitioner, Hatfield Heath, Essex.

Foreword

Health as a social good is being reaffirmed throughout the world, and in the United States health care is finally being recognized as a right rather than a privilege. Meanwhile, critical examination of the effectiveness and efficiency of health systems worldwide finds most health sectors in need of major reform. In rich and poor countries alike too much is spent on health interventions of low cost-effectiveness, such as surgical treatment of many cancers, and too little is spent on services of high cost-effectiveness such as preventive care, prenatal care and treatment of sexually transmitted diseases. More cost-effective use of scarce health resources promises to improve health outcomes for the same expenditure while offering policy-makers a rational method of choosing which services to finance.

Nowhere is the scrutiny of health systems more intense than in the United States and the United Kingdom. This timely book examines the premises upon which these two societies built their health systems and the forces that are stimulating reform efforts. Against the larger background of a global health economy of $1,700 billion (about 8% of the 1990 total world product), the USA, the UK and the remaining established market economies, with 15% of the world's population, consumed 87% of global health expenditures. The USA alone, with 5% of the population, consumed 41% of the global health budget in 1990 – almost $3,000 per person compared with $41 per person in the developing world. The UK, spending just over $1,000 per person in 1990, achieved better health outcomes and guaranteed access to care for all of its citizens.

These sharp differences between consumption in the USA and the UK reflect what the authors spell out in compelling detail – the National Health Service in the UK is based on a strong foundation of primary care, a manpower plan based on the health care needs of its citizens and a global budget, which despite the figures enumerated above is regarded as too small to meet current needs. Nonetheless, the citizens of the UK receive good care at moderate cost. The USA, on the other hand, has neither a manpower plan nor a budget; fee-for-service payments with third-party reimbursement have separated supply from demand, and the medical profession with its capacity to generate its own demand has further distorted market forces. The USA, with medical expenditures the highest in the world, health outcomes towards the lower end of the established market economies, and a system of care that rations by social class, employment and type of care – is all too often getting poor care at high cost.

Calls for reform in both countries must respond to common dilemmas. Finite resources have to be allocated more efficiently to achieve maximum health benefit for aging societies. Some restrictions will be inevitable. They should be determined by cost-effectiveness criteria, a population-based view of societal need, and appropriate research to inform ethical debate, improve manpower policies, and increase efficiency within the respective systems. As the authors emphasize, both societies will also have to rely more on individual responsibility to adopt health-promoting behaviors and social responsibility to assure fairness and equity. This book should be read by all engaged in the debate about reform of the health sector on both sides of the Atlantic.

Robert S Lawrence
Director, Health Sciences
Rockefeller Foundation
March 1994

Preface

Unashamedly this is a biased book! It is biased towards our thesis that primary care is the essential foundation for any cost-effective health care system. We believe that strong primary care leads to better care that is more satisfying, more economical and with better outcomes. It is a most important missing element in the American system, and American professionals can learn from the British. As Americans rediscover the centrality and value of primary care, the British are expanding it into new forms that increase its effectiveness. The British have already the best primary care system in the West (*see* Table 8.2), and are forging ahead with yet more improvements.

Since the 1978 WHO/UNICEF conference and its Alma Ata Declaration highlighted primary care as 'essential', there has been little co-ordinated follow-up to promote and implement its assertions. There is need now to bring together international experiences to produce model(s) of excellence for primary care and to learn from one another.

This was John Fry's last book created out of his experiences over the last 45 years as a general practitioner and as an acknowledged authority in primary care throughout the world. John Fry had also traveled widely and served at times as a WHO consultant and adviser. The book benefits from the practical experiences of Jonathan Rodnick, a US family physician and professor at the University of California, San Francisco who leads a major department of family medicine in the thick of corporate managed care; and from the overall guidance of Donald Light at the University of Medicine and Dentistry of New Jersey. We acknowledge all the support that the Rockefeller Foundation and Robert Lawrence have given to primary care and thank him for his foreword.

This book discusses the nature, features and roles of primary care in general terms and in more detail those in the US and UK. The evolution of any health system has to relate to the national history, social philosophies and attitudes, wealth, geography and political views and wishes of the people and the professionals, but there are priorities in all systems and one of these is the place and strength of primary care. After comparing the US and UK health systems we focus on primary care in the two countries and consider what each can teach the other.

The concept for this book was initiated by four recognized authorities resulting in occasional duplication of facts and a few differences in their interpretation. The publishers acknowledge these features and believe they enrich the text, providing an agenda for discussions and actions towards stronger primary care within all health systems.

Much of this book was initially written by John Fry during a Rockefeller Foundation Residency at the Villa Serbelloni, Bellagio, Italy.

Donald Light
Jonathan Rodnick
Peter Orton
March 1995

List of Abbreviations

AAFP	American Academy of Family Physicians
AMA	American Medical Association
BMA	British Medical Association
CCU	coronary care unit
COGME	Council of Graduate Medical Education
CQI	continuous quality improvement
DGH	District General Hospital
DHA	District Health Authority
ERISA	Employee Retirement Income Security Act
FHSA	Family Health Services Authority
FMG	foreign medical graduate
FP	family physician
GDP	Gross Domestic Product
GMC	General Medical Council
GMSC	General Medical Services Committee
GP	general practitioner/physician
HMO	Health Maintenance Organization
HPSA	health provision shortage area
ICU	intensive care unit
IMG	international medical graduate
IPA	Independent Practice Organization
LMC	Local Medical Committee

MPC   Medical Practices Committee

NHS   National Health Service

OTC   over the counter

PMC   Primary Managed Care

RBRVS   Resource Based Relative Value System

PPO   Preferred Provider Organization

RCGP   Royal College of General Practitioners

RHA   Rural Health Authority

WHO   World Health Organization

1

Health Care

Common Dilemmas and Responsibilities

All nations face an insoluble equation in striving to provide health care for all. Diseases will never be exterminated or prevented completely and will always need to be treated, and if not cured, relief and comfort provided. The demand for medical care is increasing with people's expectations and medical advances. There is no single best-buy system that is applicable universally but basic models of excellence should be considered.

Common dilemmas are how to allocate, share and use finite resources. Some restrictions with priorities are inevitable but should be made easier if everyone accepts personal and social responsibilities and collaboration in a planned, national health system believed to be fair and equitable. Primary care is the keystone to any health care system and is the best foundation for reducing risks and therefore illnesses. In the 21st century a tidal wave of chronicity will hit all advanced systems.

The US and UK present portraits in contrast. Both are undergoing radical reform, the UK perhaps greater than the US. But the UK is greatly strengthening and extending primary care – already the strongest in the West – while the US is elaborating complexes of specialists bundled into managed care systems. The level of technology and profit that span the American approach will lead to escalating costs and painful rationing that a more sane system would avoid. The need to understand the true character of primary care could not be more urgent.

How Much Health, Disease and Care in the Community?

Attempts to provide care for people which is efficient, effective, economic and equitable face the insoluble equation of wants being greater than needs, which in turn will always be greater than available resources. No health care system can possibly provide complete care and meet every want and need of the patient and physician, and be appropriate to all nations. Yet systems with a sound and stable knowledge of primary care are likely to come closest.

Health has been defined by the World Health Organization (WHO) foundation since 1948, as 'a state of complete physical, mental and social wellbeing and not merely an absence of disease'. Continuing health as so defined must be an unusual condition! The situation was complicated further when the WHO in 1978 produced global targets for all countries to promote Health for All: 2000. Although this is laudable, health and its attainment and maintenance are likely to remain elusive.

'Health' is a subjective and an objective state. Its WHO definition must include how people feel at anytime, how well they are able to perform their normal daily functions, what symptoms they are experiencing and what disease labels have been attached by physicians. In other words, a condition influenced by many factors. Objectively, it is difficult to create a totally composite picture of the state of health of people in any society at any one time.

In the UK a consumer study (British Market Research Bureau, 1987) reported that while 75% of those questioned considered themselves 'above average in health', 34% 'in very good health' and 39% 'fairly good', nevertheless, when presented with a checklist of 80 specified ailments, almost everyone had suffered from at least one in the past 12 months (an average of 13.3 per adult) and even in a two week period, nine out of 10 had suffered from an average of 5.5 ailments. Admittedly, most of the ailments in adults were minor; 33% reported tiredness, 33% headache, and 25% aches and pains. In children, 25% had suffered from colds and coughs and 33% from cuts, grazes or bruises.

Kohn and White (1976) found that at any time, 66% of people in the US and UK, and often in other countries, were taking medicines. Of these, 33% were prescribed and 33% self-medicated with over the counter (OTC) preparations. The following British data for an average year (1992) illustrates how extensively people use available health services (Orton and Fry, 1995):

- 80% of the population consult their family physician (GP) at least once a year

- the average patient consultation rate for a GP is 3–4 consultations per person per year

- 14% of the population is admitted to hospital

- 18% of the population is referred by their GP to a secondary care specialist (there is no self-referral in the UK)

- 23% of the population attend a hospital accident and emergency department.

Comparisons between those attending and not attending their family physician show that both groups report similar rates of minor illness. The non-attenders were much more self-reliant, managed their own problems and had a more discriminating opinion of the medical profession.

The broad spectrum of non-health and disease, ranging from mortal diseases to minor dysphoria, includes:

- *dysphoria* – a state of ill at ease and dissatisfaction with one's own situation and environment

- *sickness* – ailments suitable for self-care

- *illness* – disorders considered appropriate by patient, or family, for advice/care from a physician or other health professional

- *disease* – when a diagnostic label is applied by a physician. There are many sub-groups, identified by ICD classification, and their grade of severity, prognosis and functional disability

- *death* – cause certified by a physician.

Within UK primary care, the proportions of disease seen in general practice are:

- *minor ailments* – self-limiting and benign (46% of consultations in the UK)

- *chronic (mental and physical) disorders* – associated with aging and producing long-term functional disability and need for care (40% of consultations)

- *major diseases* – life-threatening and often acute, requiring collaboration between many physicians and facilities. For example, heart and stroke emergencies, cancers, accidents and major infections (14% of consultations).

In addition, and of considerable relevance in caring for people and understanding their predicaments, are the social problems and pathologies in a community. The impact of social problems makes the achievement of the WHO health targets even less likely, and the differences and inequalities in health status between upper and lower social groups in all countries urgently need addressing.

Traditional measurements of the causes and extent of morbidity and mortality, plus indices of quality such as infant mortality rates, life expectancies and rates of chronic and disabling disorders, provide gross information at macro levels. More sophisticated, detailed measurements are necessary to provide data on outcomes of care in relation to various forms of management and their cost benefits. In planning the utilization of limited resources it is important to know which preventive, therapeutic and diagnostic procedures are useful and effective, and which should be discouraged and even prohibited and which individuals and groups are at particular risk. In the future, measures of effective care are likely to become increasingly important.

With health care, in spite of advances in medical sciences and technologies, we can still only endeavor to:

Cure sometimes

Relieve often

Comfort always

Prevent if possible.

The inevitability of disease and non-health means that we must apply the science of the possible and the art of the impossible. We have to make use of available resources for the greatest common good. A good health care system must acknowledge and understand the many factors involved in causation and prevalence of non-health and disease, in addition to biomedical causes. These could be summarized as shown below.

- *Personal* – lifestyle, including smoking, alcohol and drug misuse, overweight, nutrition, exercise, and genetic family factors, not only are some diseases inherited but there are many excess predispositions and liabilities to poor health which may relate to family.

- *Social and environmental* – the social factors underlying the prevalence, course and outcome of many different diseases are influenced by: wealth/poverty, housing, nutrition, (un)employment, occupational hazards, crime, national and local policies, environment (physical and social).

The WHO Health for All: 2000 directive implies that health care is a human right. However, limits need to be acknowledged and sensitive questions posed.

Faced with the insoluble equation of health care, decisions have to be made on how much care can be provided within a nation's resources. Priorities and rationing are inevitable, but who is to decide on them and on what basis? What care, for whom and by whom? Responsibilities of all those involved – public, professionals, providers and politicians – have to be defined, accepted and applied.

Primary care is a vehicle for teaching acceptance of chronic problems, management skills, support skills, techniques for risk reduction. It is a Partnership for Health. For all there are common dilemmas. Faced with apparently infinite demands on finite resources, attempts to provide health services come up against not only limits in funding but limitations in the potential of even the most modern technology to resolve problems of ill health and disease. Sooner or later this leads to inevitable insufficiencies and the need for priorities in the allocation of resources, or 'rationing'.

The dilemmas then are how best to provide health care for people that is efficient, effective, economic, equitable, and at the same time is accessible, available, acceptable, appreciated, appropriate, affordable, achievable and accountable. Since health care is a human right and expectation, everyone must accept some responsibility for creating the best possible model for its delivery.

Responsibilities, Roles and Power

There are four main groups with roles and responsibilities for health care provision:

- *politicians (lay and medical)*
- *providers and purchasers (managers)*
- *professionals (clinicians)*
- *patients (the people)*.

Politicians

In democracies, politicians are the elected representatives of the people who serve in national or local government, supported by a collection of bureaucrats, civil servants and others. There are ministries and departments for health and welfare at various levels.

The role of politicians should be as visionaries and leaders, developing policies and defining the broad principles which form the basis of universal systems of health care. They should be responsible for making decisions on how the national health system should be organized, for estimating the likely resources which will be required, for defining standards and quality of services provided and for establishing possible checks and controls on health care delivery. Their plans and decisions have to be based on accurate and reliable data and information, and a data collection service must be in operation at all levels.

Politicians need to realize that good health is only partly dependent on medical services. It is more closely related to environmental and social conditions in the community, and to family and individual conditions. They should be concerned with the care of those weaker and disadvantaged members of society and with preventive measures, as well as with the implementation of the latest modern medical technologies.

Politicians should be sensitive also to public concerns, complaints, expectations and wants, because their re-election may depend on the quality of health care in their constituencies. However decisions influenced by the public may be popular but not make the best use of resources. One has to remember that not all wants and needs can be met.

Managers

Providers vary with the system. Thus, they may be part of a government national health system; they may be part of a health insurance system; they may be private entrepreneurs or employees of medical faculties providing personal care (physicians, nurses etc), or resources and facilities, such as hospitals or diagnostic services.

Whatever the scheme, someone somewhere has to pay for it and this may be through:

- taxation that is either general or health care specific
- prepaid health insurance schemes which may be part of a national non-profit social insurance program or private competitive for-profit businesses
- out-of-pocket payments, either by total fees-for-services or as additional partial co-payments for services, drugs or other arrangements
- charities for specific small groups
- a combination of all or some of these.

Providers' roles and responsibilities are as administrators, managers and organizers of health services. They may be civil servants, private organization employees, or self-employed. In the UK, they manage facilities which provide services and are not usually fund-raisers, but they are responsible for allocated budgets which in theory, should not be over-run. In practice, this is well nigh impossible. They are concerned with getting value for money and must rely on good financial and operational data. All this requires certain controls and checks on quality and quantity which may not be popular with professionals and the public. Although rarely achievable, providers should collaborate closely with politicians, professionals and the public at various levels. In the UK the medical profession is increasingly becoming managed.

Clinicians

The clinicians are the 'carers'; their roles are to provide care and service to individuals and communities to the highest possible standards, but within limitations of resources. The greater medical profession includes physicians, nurses and other health workers.

As professionals, they are a select and privileged group in society with lengthy training and acceptance of standards, ethics and morals that are controlled in various ways. The medical profession has a high status and image, with incomes many times the national average and with considerable power and influence in health care planning and management. The profession maintains ethics and protects and monitors standards of health care. It has cherished 'clinical freedom' but now this has to be adapted to responsibilities for achieving outcomes in terms of efficient, effective and economic care coupled with checks, controls and audits to avoid useless procedures and therapies (Hoffenberg, 1987).

These professionals may work as private, independent entrepreneurs or as salaried employees. They may work from their own premises and with their own equipment, or from facilities such as hospitals or clinics owned by others. Their motivation may be professional, but they are also influenced by pay, rewards, incentives and competition. Care is also provided by non-professional carers. These are family friends and informal networks who provide the backup for ancillary services and without whose dedication no system can function. These carers also need to be cared for and supported.

People

The people (the public) are the ultimate payers, through various paymasters of taxation, insurance, or out-of-pocket fees. There is nothing 'free' in medical care – even charitable institutions have to be funded. There is concern everywhere at rising costs of medical care, no matter whether these costs are to be met by higher taxes or by rising insurance premiums, or by out-of-pocket direct or co-payments.

Since people know that they are paying for health services, they are increasingly keen to have their rights, wants, needs, and expectations attended to! However, these basic wants and expectations are not inappropriate. In general terms, they are:

- good quality care with good results

- comprehensive coverage of care for themselves and their families

- available and accessible first-contact and long-term services

- personal service and attention with human kindness, concern and sensitivity

- appropriate (but not excessive) care, including diagnosis and treatment as well as avoidance of unnecessary procedures involving discomfort and pain

- adequate time with physician, including explanation and information and shared decision-making

- some freedom of choice of physician and services

- opportunities to complain and receive redress.

However, the individual and family have their own responsibilities in using available services with discrimination and without excess; accepting the need for self-care, self-reliance, health promotion and maintenance, and applying accepted principles of prevention.

Adequate preventive care includes:

- immunization, screening and counselling

- timely access to diagnostic and specialized care

- emergency services

- hospitalization when needed

- long-term community care

- public health and environmental services.

Ultimately, the best system and the best services will be achieved through collaboration and understanding of all our responsibilities. In other words, politicians are people who must be concerned for their fellows and managers must be closely involved with them, as well as with clinicians and the public. In turn clinicians cannot exist without political support, without provision of facilities or resources, and without people as patients. People should be involved at and with all the other levels.

Essential to understanding the realities, limitations and limits of a national health care organization is a sound national education system and wide spread information through news media, who must accept their own responsibilities for accuracy and avoidance of over expectations.

Summary

Health is a utopian mirage, with few people being completely healthy for any length of time. Most illnesses are minor and self-limiting, and make up over one-half of primary care practice. One-third are chronic and long-term and about two-thirds are major and life-threatening problems. The spectrum of non-health ranges from dysphoria through sickness, illness, disease and disability, to death.

There is an insoluble equation to health care with wants and needs always exceeding available resources, and this means priorities and rationing. Limitations, even of modern medicine, must be understood by all – we can only 'cure sometimes, relieve often, comfort always, and prevent if possible'.

The challenges are to employ the science of the possible with the art of the impossible and to provide a service as efficient, economic and as equitable as possible. We need to decide how to best meet these insufficiencies and who will make the decisions.

The responsibilities of health care have to be shared by all. Politicians act as elected representatives of the people and must take decisions on policies at national and local levels. Providers and purchasers act as administrators, managers and fund allocators and must ensure good value for money. Professionals in the greater medical profession, and other carers, are trained in modern sciences and technologies; but they have to combine this with sensitive, personal care and service – recognizing that their actions may be influenced by payments, rewards and incentives.

People have to realize that health care is never free and has to be paid for – by them ultimately – but they must also have a guaranteed contract of basic rights for good, available and accessible care for all with appropriate, but not excessive, professional management to meet individual needs.

An efficient, effective, economic and equitable health system demands full collaboration between all these groups with strong, sensible and sensitive leadership.

2

Health Care Systems: an International Overview

Introduction

All health systems face similar problems of rising costs, increasing aging and dependent populations with fewer younger carers, and escalating costs of new forms of medical treatment and technology. The challenges of achieving best values for health care monies is shared by all – the current popular philosophy is 'competitive marketing through managed care' and we strive to learn from each other. There are similarities and differences.

Each nation has its own historical roots and beliefs that are transmitted to the philosophies of a health system. All involve public–private mixes of different proportions. There are differences in costs by percentage of Gross Domestic Product (GDP) and per capita expenditures, intensity of use of diagnostic and therapeutic procedures, population coverage and public satisfactions.

There are four levels of care in every system (Figure 2.1). The roles of and relations between primary and secondary professional services are particularly important. Costs, cover, satisfaction and health indices rates are related to the strengths of primary care services in the national systems. With so many common problems and dilemmas in the provision of national health care, it is instructive to compare how different countries are coping, and with what degree of success.

Increasing public expectations of health and disease care lead to demands for the latest and most modern services. Coupled with the demographic changes of low birth and low fertility rates and longer life expectancies, with aging and dependent populations inevitably requiring more care. Business efficiency and market management principles are being applied in the hope of getting the best possible value for money out of a profession that has until now put care before profit. The consequence of these attitudes has been: closure of hospital beds and in-patient services, transference to out-patient ambulatory and day-care procedures, more demands for care from community-based services and a new look at generalist primary care, and its potentials for saving costs by accepting more tasks and roles and acting as gatekeepers or gateopeners to, and protectors of, more expensive and specialist services. However, accepting that evidence may

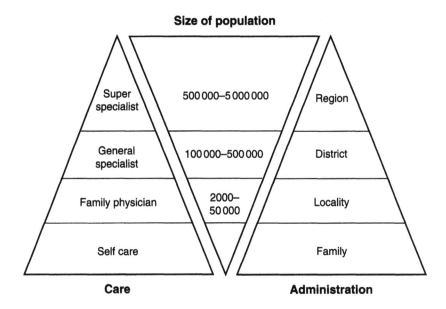

Figure 2.1   Levels of Care, Population and Administration.

be forthcoming, so far there is little to suggest that these changes can lead to lower expenditures.

When comparing different systems of health care, a check list is helpful (Fry and Horder, 1993) and consists of:

- *national characteristics*
- *system of health care*
- *structure and levels of care*
- *services and processes*
- *outcomes*
- *public satisfaction.*

National Characteristics

The shape of health and socio-economic systems is strongly influenced by: national philosophies (cultural and religious principles); wealth and economic systems (the wealthier a nation, the more it spends on health care); geography, population density and infrastructure; demography (eg birth rates, population growth); social problems, community attitudes; political decisions.

Table 2.1 Expenditure on health services by percentage of GDP

Health service location	GDP (percentage)
USA	over 14
France The Netherlands Sweden	8–9
UK Japan Denmark	5–7

The expenditures on health services by percentage of GDP are shown in Table 2.1.

Demographic details give some indication, but need to be combined with other indicators such as GDP per head and trading successes etc. The demographic details shown in Table 2.2 are similar in developed countries.

Systems

Gradual evolution of health care systems has always been more successful in countries with stable social systems than radical revolution. Some government funding is necessary to meet basic levels of care.

Few people can afford to pay directly for the costs of major disease care and procedures. In response, Western, affluent countries based on capitalist economies, vary greatly in the degree to which they fund care for public sources (Table 2.1). All except the US made access to medical services a right of citizenship long ago and therefore use public funding extensively. Most of the public funds in the US go to services for the poor and elderly, that are inflated by an essentially private insurance system.

Few private insurance schemes can meet all the health care needs, for example, long-term and community care for chronic physical and mental diseases, care of the aged and severely disabled.

The main types of health care systems are:

- comprehensive national health and social security as in the UK and Sweden paid largely out of taxation

- non-profit but government supervised social security and health insurance paid out of employer–employee contributions plus public (government) funding as in France, Germany, The Netherlands, Japan, Denmark and Canada

Table 2.2 Demographic indices for selected countries (Fry and Horder, 1994; *The Economist*, 1992)

Country	Under 15	Over 65	Birth rate per 1,000	Fertility rate per woman	Infant mortality per 1,000 births	Life expectancy M	F
USA	21.4	12.6	14.1	1.9	9.0	73	80
UK	19.0	15.4	13.7	1.8	7.4	73	79
Canada	20.9	11.4	12.9	1.7	7.3	74	81
Japan	18.4	11.7	11.5	1.7	6.0	76	82
Germany	16.0	14.9	10.9	1.5	7.5	73	79
France	20.1	13.8	13.4	1.8	7.5	73	81
Sweden	17.3	18.1	12.6	1.9	5.7	75	81

- private insurance schemes with some public funding for special social groups as in the US

- a mix of private insurance for affluent and public for poor as in Hong Kong and Singapore.

The proportions of public funding for all health services range from almost total coverage to under 50%:

- US: 40–50%

- Japan, Australia, Germany, France, and UK: 75–90%

- Sweden, socialist countries and oil-rich countries: over 90%.

Table 2.3 Annual percentage of GDP spent on health care (public and private) and annual per capita expenditure (US$) (OHE, 1992)

Country	Annual GDP% expenditure (1990–1) Public (%)	Private (%) (US$)	Total	Annual per capital expenditure US$	£
USA	5.2 (42)	7.2 (58)	12.4	3,200	2,133
UK	5.2 (85)	0.9 (15)	6.1	1,097	731
Canada	6.7 (75)	2.3 (25)	9.0	1,825	1,217
Japan	4.9 (75)	1.6 (25)	6.5	1,652	1,101
Germany	5.9 (73)	2.2 (27)	8.1	1,863	1,242
France	6.6 (74)	2.3 (26)	8.9	1,750	1,167
Sweden	7.8 (90)	0.9 (10)	8.7	2,300	1,533

Table 2.4 Populations per physician and annual new medical graduates (Fry and Horder, 1994)

Country	Population per physician	% Women physicians	Population per primary physicians	Population per annual medical graduates
US	440	18	1,365	15,600
Sweden	330	28	2,430	15,000
Germany	354	27	1,067	4,571
Japan	610	10	1,600	14,750
Canada	491	20	1,152	15,360
France	333	27	1,120	16,000
UK	575	26	1,742	15,000

Proportion of Public Expenditure Spent on Health Care

The considerable variations in the rates of population per physician and annual numbers of new medical graduates suggest uncertainties in medical manpower requirements (Table 2.4).

The different rates of population per primary physician suggest differences in policy priorities. There are almost twice as many physicians per head of population in France and Sweden as in Japan; twice the population per primary physician in Sweden as in Canada, Germany and France. It is difficult to compare 'primary physicians' per head of population because of differing definitions, here we take the broadest definition of a 'first-contact' physician.

The high output of medical graduates in Germany is related to laws which do not allow restricted entry into medical schools. In countries with an excess of doctors for their requirements, this may result in the migration to other countries or unemployment within their own country. Medical manpower resources need to be planned and include the number of doctors going through medical schools. All these differences occur with similar outcomes of care.

Comparing the UK and US the number of population per physician is similar. In addition in the US about 5,000 international medical graduates are admitted, but in the UK permanent medical immigration is only 600 (Table 2.5).

The annual mean growth rates per 100,000 is 2–5 for the two nations, meaning additional physicians of 6,000 in the US and 1,500 in the UK. Are all these extra physicians really necessary? (Table 2.6)

Table 2.5 Primary physicians in the US and UK in rates per 100,000 (1963–1990) and average annual changes in rates per 100,000 and numbers (JRSM, 1994)

	USA				UK
Per 100,000 population	All primary physicians	Family physicians	General internists	General pediatricians	GP
1963	57	34	16	7	44
1990	87	28	42	17	59
Annual change per 100,000	+ 1.0	− 0.2	+ 1.0	+ 0.3	+ 0.6
Annual change in total numbers of physicians	+ 2,750	− 500	+ 2,500	+ 750	+ 315

Table 2.6 Physicians providing direct patient care per 100,000 in the US and UK during 1963 and 1992 (JRSM, 1994)

	Number of physicians per 100,000		Ratios		
Year	US	UK	US		UK
1963	135	81	1.7	:	1
1992	204	160	1.3	:	1
Annual growth	2.38	2.72			

What is a 'Primary Physician'?

The four, functional levels of care in every health care system are:

- *self care*
- *primary generalist professional care*
- *secondary specialist care*
- *tertiary specialist care.*

When a person decides to seek professional care in the UK and US, there are differences; in the UK the individual has direct access to an NHS general practitioner (GP), while in the US the person has access to any physician (Figure 2.2).

Whoever he or she is, the primary physician has similar roles and functions in the US and UK. These are to provide direct access, first-contact assessment, decisions on management and whether referral to other secondary specialists is necessary.

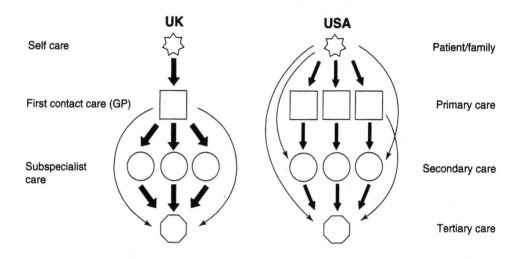

Figure 2.2 Flow of Care for UK and US Health Systems.

In the UK, the primary physician is the 'general practitioner'; an independent contractor with the NHS, not a salaried employee. He enters into contract to provide comprehensive care for patients who 'register' with him. He is paid in a mix of capitation and other fees with reimbursements and other methods. The GP is the gatekeeper to specialist services. He provides care for all ages and works in a team and with community services.

In the US, the situation is more complex. The patients play the role of being their own GP; they decide which specialists to see and when and this decision is based on their perceived need. There are no statutory responsibilities for comprehensive care and each physician works to his own rules and ethics. Thus, the American citizen can consult any physician at first contact. In the US, the nearest equivalents to the British GP are family physicians or practitioners who provide care for families and all ages. The other three kinds of 'primary care' doctors have a notably narrower range, these are:

- *general internists* who provide medical care to adults but often not psychiatric or surgical services

- *general pediatricians* who care for children

- *general obstetricians/gynecologists* who care for women.

As noted, persons can also consult at first-contact any secondary or tertiary specialists. As such, there are definite gatekeeping roles, but referrals between these generalists and specialists are common. Table 2.7 shows comparisons and contrasts between the US and UK.

Table 2.7 Comparisons between UK and US primary physicians

UK: General practitioner	US: Primary physician
• Statutory responsibilities for registered patients • Direct access – availability on 24 hour basis • Oversee long-term comprehensive care • Gatekeeping roles (strict) • Responsibility for primary care teams • Shared care with specialists • Community responsibilities • No direct access to specialists	• Family physicians – care for all ages and have some gatekeeping roles • General internists – care for common problems of adults • General pediatricians – general, preventive and specialist care for children • General OBG – direct access care for women • Specialists – of any type and grade, usually transient care for specific problems • Direct access to specialists

The Funding of Health Care

There are four methods of paying for health care (Chapter 1, p. 6), and in many systems there exist combinations of a public–private mix.

1. Out-of-pocket payments by individuals exist in all systems. They range from total payments for some excluded services such as dental treatment, physiotherapy and psychotherapy, to cost-sharing and partner payments as a proportion of the fees. For example, in the US an insurance policy may require the patient to pay the first $1,000, for a percentage of the total bill, or fixed amounts of the physician's fees and medication. In most systems there are some user payments for prescribed drugs, but specified, essential, life-saving drugs are usually free. There may be user payments for proportions of physicians' fees for services and some token payment for hospital 'hotel services' or standard day charges.

2. The system most widely used is prepaid, medical (health) insurance, in which those involved pay regular premiums into a common pool, large enough to pay for certain agreed services. There are various national insurance schemes.

    • *Voluntary schemes* – do not cover the whole population and are usually part of employment conditions, with contributions from employers and employees. Additional arrangements have to be made for the uninsured.

- *Compulsory national insurance schemes* – the whole of a population are contributors and beneficiaries. Within such schemes there may be a number of programs, eg for workers, the self-employed and the retired.

- *For-profit health insurance companies* – middle-men between the insured person and the provider. Their roles are to collect premiums and to make arrangements with providers for rates of fees for services.

- *Quasi-government social insurance agencies* – do not make a profit and are independent of government, also acting as middle-men.

3. National health systems are part of a government public service, with all the health services under the direction of a government department or ministry. There are differing arrangements with hospitals and physicians, with either or both having variable degrees of independence. Thus, physicians are not necessarily government employees.

4. In all systems there is back-up from charity organizations. For example, the development of the hospice movement.

Paying Physicians

Within any system a major influencing factor on the services provided is the way in which physicians are paid. Whatever the system, the possible methods of physician remuneration are:

- *open fees for services* – the levels being decided by the physician and or medical organization

- *controlled fees for services* – in many insurance schemes the physician receives a set fee for specified services, usually at a lower level than 'open' fees

- *capitation fees* – agreed fees paid for by persons who are 'registered' with a physician, the fee is paid whether the patient is well and does not consult, or sick; when any number of consultations may be made. In capitation schemes, there may be extra fees paid to physicians for specific services, such as preventive procedures, minor surgery, check-ups, etc.

- *salaried physicians* – may work in hospitals or in primary care and this scheme may be part of a national health system, as in Sweden or the UK for hospital specialists, or a Health Maintenance Organization (HMO) in the US.

Structure

Within every system there are four recognizable and essential levels related to care, population size and administration mentioned earlier (Figure 2.1). Each level has its own roles and requires its own training, facilities and resources, and each has to relate and collaborate with the other levels.

1. *Self care* in a family context, with responsibilities for care of minor ailments.

2. *Primary care* where it is providing access to personal, first-contact care, and long-term continuing family care over the years in a population of around 2,000 per primary physician. The conditions encountered are the common minor, chronic and major diseases in a population of that size, ie 2,000. Secondary care implies a degree of specialization and expertise one up from primary care. Where closed referral systems operate (eg Western Europe, Canada, Australia and New Zealand), secondary specialists deal with those problems referred to them by primary physicians. Their work content will be preselected by the latter. For example, a UK GP will encounter three cases of acute appendicitis a year in his practice of 2,000 patients, while the general surgeons at the local district general hospital (population base 250,000) will operate on 375 cases referred to them by 125 GPs (*see also* Chapter 6). In addition to general clinical duties, the physician has some responsibility for the social and preventive care of the local community and in acting as co-ordinator, protector and decision-maker to more complex specialist services (*see also* Chapters 5 and 6).

    In the organization of family physicians, trends in the UK have been towards groups of GPs working within a health team. The mean size of a UK general practice unit is five GPs. In the UK only 1 in 10 are solo, whereas in the US this is 1 in 3 (Table 2.8).

3. *Secondary general specialist care*, appropriate in a district general hospital serving a population of around 250,000. The specialists, who may be hospital or office based, are general physician-internists, general surgeons,

Table 2.8 Percentage of family physicians (US) and general practitioners (UK) working in groups of different sizes (RSM, 1994)

Group size	US (%)	UK (%)
Solo	37	11
Two partners	13	15
Three/four partners	–	36
Five or more partners	33	17
Multi-specialty	17	21

general obstetricians and gynecologists, general pediatricians, general psychiatrists, general orthopedists etc.

4. *Tertiary subspecialist care*, based on regions serving between 1 and 5 million people associated with academic centers for high technology services, eg investigations and surgery, neuroradiology, and pediatric intensive care.

Services and Processes

The basic services provided are similar in all health care systems. They are a combination of accepted professional methods and customs, coupled with attempts to meet increasing public demands and expectations for rights of care.

In developed societies the prevalent clinical problems are very similar (*see also* Chapters 5 and 6), although the mix, and particularly the social problems, differ not only between countries but also between regions and districts. For example, in the US the trend has been for increased specialization and the use of technology, whereas in the UK, more prominence has been given to primary medical care and community care. One example of this has been the large expenditure on modern hospitals in the US and the relative neglect of hospital rebuilding in the UK, where many buildings are over 50 years old.

In the flow of care the primary physician occupies an important role. As the first professional contact he or she has to make decisions as to whether the patient can be managed at the primary level or needs to be referred to other specialists. With pressures in the UK to carry out more at the primary level, including health promotion, and refer fewer patients to specialists, the processes of care are changing, and so is the organization. In the US, patients have direct access to secondary care specialists, and the gatekeeper role of primary care physicians is not established. In the US, fear of litigation is leading to greater pressures towards defensive measures including questionable reasons for investigations and referrals to subspecialists.

There are wide differences between the UK and US in a number of areas. For example the cesarean section rates are 25% of births in the US and 12% in the UK. Expenditure on medication was $110 per capita in the US and £64 in the UK in 1992.

Solo practice is declining and more physicians are working in groups of generalists or multi-specialty groups. Primary health teams are developing with increasing roles for nurses and other paramedical professionals working with generalist and specialist physicians. The accent on efficiency, effectiveness and economics is leading to a much more business orientated re-organization with management involvements, audits and attention to implementing more useful procedures and cutting down on unproven, ineffective ones. In the UK this has led to the introduction of fund (budget) holding among general practices (Chapter 6).

Table 2.9 Weekly volume of patient–physician contacts in the US and UK (JRSM, 1994)

Site	US	UK
Office	108	109
Hospital	17	–
Nursing home	7	–
Home visit	2	19
Total	134	128

Table 2.10 Weekly hours in direct patient care in the US and UK (family physicians and general practitioners) (JRSM, 1994)

Contact	US (h)	UK (h)
Direct patient care	48.4	37.01
Other	7.8	5.0 (plus 23.50 'on call')
Total	56.2	42.01

The annual person consultation rates for ambulatory primary care are 3.0 in the US and 3.3 in the UK.

The *weekly volume of direct* patient–physician contacts (Table 2.9) is higher and more widely distributed in the US.

The *weekly working times* for US family physicians (FP) and UK GPs (Table 2.10) show that US physicians have a longer working week in direct contact with patients and their consultation times (12–13 min.) are longer than in the UK (8–10 min.).

Outcomes

It is paradoxical that despite the many different systems in the various countries, the crude measurable demographic and health outcomes are similar. The differences that can be detected are related more to social and economic conditions than to any special features of the system. Thus, the health indices, such as life expectancies, infant mortality rates, birth rates, death rates and main causes of death are very similar (Table 2.2). However, there are differences in costs and satisfaction rates. The expenditures on health services by percentage of GDP vary and in the US are twice that of the UK.

Public Satisfaction

Starfield (1992), in a detailed analysis relating to health indications, cost expenditure, public satisfaction and primary care, shows a general concordance between the strength of primary care and health indicators, which also relate to public satisfaction. There was less relationship to health expenditure as a percentage of GDP.

Highest satisfaction to cost ratios were in The Netherlands and Canada, medium UK, Sweden and Germany and lowest by more than ten fold in the US. The UK, with a 'primary care score' of 1.7 and satisfaction/expense index of 2.1, compared with the US at 0.2 and 0.2, respectively.

Whilst Japan was not included in Starfield's report, it has a relatively low percentage of GDP expenditure and good health indices (Tables 2.3 and 2.6) but poor public satisfaction with health services and poor primary care (Fry and Horder, 1993).

Summary

All health systems face similar problems with increasing demands for limited resources. The cost of health care in the US is double that of the UK with apparently no improvement in measurable income. Indeed public satisfaction with health care appears to be lower in the US and in the UK was strongly associated with the strength of primary care.

A strong primary care level in a health care system offers widespread access and availability to the people with control of the use of secondary care through acting as a gatekeeper.

In any system, inefficient and ineffective practices need to be identified.

3

The UK Health Care System

Introduction

Although the British National Health Service (NHS) was set up in 1948, its roots stretch back almost 100 years. It is an established and popular part of the national social structure and provides health cover for the whole population. It is funded largely through public taxation and is one of the 'cheapest' as measured by percentage of GDP and per capital expenditure.

The UK health system costs 6% of GDP, or $1,100 per head in 1992. The number of physicians per population is a quarter less than the US at 1 physician per 600 population. The ratio of primary physician to population is lower than in the US but is evenly distributed with clearly defined roles.

There are divisions in the NHS – hospital (subspecialist), general practice (primary care generalist) and public health (community) services. All are under control of the Government Department of Health with a Secretary of State as its head and who is responsible to Parliament. The hospital services are administered by Regional and District Health Authorities (RHAs and DHAs) and the subspecialists are salaried employees of the NHS. General practice is administered by Family Health Services Authorities (FHSAs) and general practitioners (GPs) are independent contractors who contract to provide direct access and continuing primary care services to registered patients. They act as gatekeepers to subspecialists in a traditionally controlled referral system. Public community health is a mix of NHS and social, local community services and there is loose collaboration between these three parts of the health system.

Currently, 60% of NHS expenditure is on hospitals, 20% on general practice and 20% on public health (OHE, 1992). Of the 100,000 physicians, 20% are hospital subspecialists (consultants), 33% are GP principles, 40% are in training in various fields and 7% in public health. Medical manpower has been increasing by 1.5% (1,500) annually over the past decade.

Under the present Conservative Government a major reorganization took place in 1990 with the introduction of competitive internal marketing involving purchasers and providers. Present problems include relations between Government and physicians, delays for some specialist services and effects of recent reorganization.

Further changes in the management of the NHS are taking place with the abolition of regional health authorities, the merger of DHAs and FHSAs into Health Commissions or boards and the restructuring of the NHS management executive. These changes will result in the reduction of NHS management with the release of more money for direct patient care.

The Nation

The United Kingdom comprises England, Wales, Scotland and Northern Ireland – Great Britain is England, Wales and Scotland.

The UK is an old country still creating new roles. Its oldest hospital, St Bartholomew's, London, was founded 850 years ago, and primary care existed well before then. In the past 50 years the UK has passed from giving up one of the world's greatest empires to being an offshore island partner in the European Community with consequent decline in economic wealth and influence.

However, its social and welfare roots are long and strong and the NHS occupies an essential place in its medical and political fabric. Within the mother of parliaments, democracy and equality have been prominent goals, but with the logical acceptance that inequalities have always existed, and will continue, between social classes in respect to wealth and health. Ever since the first documentation of history there has been evidence of concern for the sick poor, first by the Church, who provided shelter and hospices, and for the past couple of centuries as responsibilities of local communities.

The UK has a population of 57.5 million, which is relatively static, crowded into a relatively small area where communications and transport ensure that everyone has access to public facilities, including health care. The percentage of elderly (over 65) is increasing with a decline in those under 40, resulting in an increasing dependency rate. The multi-ethnic groups make up 5.5% of the population, with India-Pakistan at 2.6%. Immigration and emigration have become low and will probably remain so. The UK is now 19th in the world wealth table by annual GDP per capita – now $16,700. The US is 9th with $25,560, Switzerland is 1st with $33,515 (Table 3.1). It is also helpful at this stage to present a table with comparative facts on the UK and US (Table 3.2). In comparing the two systems, the population growth is three times greater in the US. The proportion of elderly (over 65) are similar at 12–15%, the birth rate and infant mortality rates are similar but the cesarean section rate is 2.5 times greater in the US. Legal abortions are over double in the US.

Origins of the Health Care System

The evolution of the NHS began in the 1850s with the formation of Sick Clubs during the Industrial Revolution in the poorer areas – they were set up locally

Table 3.1 Annual GDP per capita (*The Economist*, 1994)

GDP per head	$	£
1 Switzerland	33,515	22,343
2 Luxembourg	30,950	20,633
3 Japan	26,919	17,946
4 Bermuda	26,600	17,733
5 Sweden	25,487	16,991
6 Finland	24,396	16,264
7 Norway	24,151	16,100
8 Denmark	23,676	15,784
9 USA	25,560	17,040
10 Iceland	22,362	14,908
11 Canada	21,254	14,196
12 Germany	21,248	14,165
13 France	20,603	13,735
14 Austria	20,379	13,586
15 UAE	20,131	13,420
16 Belgium	19,295	12,863
17 Italy	18,576	12,384
18 The Netherlands	18,565	12,376
19 UK	16,748	11,165
20 Australia	16,595	11,063

Table 3.2 Comparative demographic data for UK and US

	UK	US
Population (million)	57.5	250
(annual growth)	(0.3%)	(1%)
Population		
under 15	18.9%	21.4%
over 65	15.5%	12.6%
Birth rate		
annual per 1,000 population	13.4	14.1
caesarean section rate per births	10%	25%
infant mortality per 1,000 births	8.4	9.0
Legal abortions		
per 1,000 women	11.7	28.0

and individually as small, prepaid insurance schemes for workers and their families (Fry, 1988).

The principle of prepaid medical insurance was formalized in 1911 by a government act creating National Health Insurance for all workers below a certain wage level. Those covered could then 'register' with an approved general practitioner who would receive 'capitation' payments to provide general medical services. The families and dependents were not covered and had to pay fees for services.

In 1942 during the darkest days (for the UK) of World War II, Sir William Beveridge, a retired civil servant, produced a report on a model of a future welfare state which included a National Health Service for everyone. The publication of the report and its distribution to all military service personnel, as well as to all households, was a tremendous morale boost.

In 1945 in a general election the Conservative Party, under Sir Winston Churchill, was defeated by the Labour Party who had included a National Health Service in its electoral manifesto. In 1946 the NHS Act was passed and on July 5, 1948 the NHS came into being. Aneurin Bevan was the Minister of Health, a fiery Welshman, who had to overcome antagonism of the powerful British Medical Association (BMA) and a majority of physicians.

Under the NHS, all hospitals were nationalized (this was not difficult because they had in fact been so during the War 1939–45). The change for general practice was undramatic, it involved extension of the established national health insurance principles to the whole population who were able to register with a GP of their choice, who would receive capitation and other fees to provide 'all necessary general medical services' including referral to NHS specialists when necessary. An important consequence of the NHS was that GPs were separated and excluded from privileges of caring for their patients in the NHS hospitals. All hospital specialists became salaried NHS employees, but GPs retained, and still do so, an independent contractual relationship with the NHS.

In retrospect, it is amusing to note that a fundamental belief of the architects of the new NHS was that its provisions would lead to better health and fall in health expenditure! In the 1950s the annual per capita NHS expenditure was £6 ($10). In 1993 it was over £600 ($1,000). In spite of difficulties, the NHS has become an integral part of British life, well liked and respected by the public, and free at point of delivery, and no political party would dream of privatization. The 1990 reorganization attempts internal structural changes without interfering with services. A major NHS achievement has been the equal distribution of well trained specialists in every UK hospital – although one half of hospital buildings still are pre-1914!

There have also been great advances in general practice. In the 1950s most GPs worked single-handed and standards tended to be low. Gradually through professional self-motivation, including a vibrant Royal College of General Practitioners (RCGP) and negotiated changes between profession and government, general practice now is first career choice of medical students, with expanded independent group practices with health teams, and most recently, using large allocated budgets to purchase specialist services.

The distribution of GPs has been controlled for the last forty years, through the Medical Practices Committee. They are responsible for allowing new GPs to enter the NHS and have aimed to achieve equal distribution by list size. In 1952, 44% of areas were under-doctored and in 1991 this was down to 5%.

The Structure

As noted before there are four levels of care, self care, primary care, sub-specialist care and superspecialist care (Figure 2.1, p. 11). In the NHS these levels have generally corresponded to:

- individuals and households (self-care)

- Family Health Services Authorities (FHSAs) administering general practice (primary care). Fundholding has been introduced over the last few years and in 1995 is extended to cover 50% of the UK population, with 1,500 funds involving 10,500 GPs. Fundholding enables a practice to be responsible for their own budget to purchase care for patients. The budget includes staff, prescribing, some investigations and referrals to secondary care and will be expanded to include community and other secondary care services. The practices can use savings to further improve facilities

- District Health Authorities (DHAs) responsible for subspecialty district general hospital services (general specialist secondary care). More recently, some hospitals have become NHS Trusts. These secondary care units are not under the control of the DHA but the Department of Health through the NHS management. Each trust is a directly managed provider unit free to market their services. The trusts provide health care services to pur-chasers' specifications, manage delivery to quantity and cost targets set in contracts, and are financially controlled

- Regional Health Authorities (RHAs). RHAs act as agents of the health secretary in the administration of the health service. Their role is the imple-mentation of national policies in the region, the DHAs and the FHSAs, resource allocation and performance monitoring, fundholding control and regulating the purchaser-provider relationships. They also have responsi-bility for superspeciality services (tertiary care)

- Department of Health (DoH) in overall control of policies, funding and services and responsible to Parliament and the people (national policies).

The Services

The NHS system allows an easy, effective, efficient and economic flow of care to be provided for all persons according to their needs.

The GP, as the personally chosen doctor for each patient, is a single entry point into the NHS (apart from hospital emergency services). There is 24-hour access and availability to a GP for all patients. In his or her contract with the NHS the GP agrees to provide all necessary general medical services to his or her patients round the clock; if not personally, he or she is responsible for arranging cover – this is shared with partners of neighboring practices. In such a scheme it is possible to incorporate gatekeeping roles for GPs.

In the UK an accepted and defined referral system to specialists existed even before the NHS (1948). Thus, in the UK patients do not have direct access to a specialist (it is unethical for a specialist to see a patient without referral from a GP, on the grounds that the specialist should be clinically supervised by a patient's primary care physician). The GP has to provide a referral letter or report to a specialist with his or her patient and the specialist has to refer the patient back to the GP with a report on completion of services. This ethical process of a GP referring to a specialist also occurs in the private sector. Some specialists in the private sector provide direct access to secondary care for the patients, undermining the gatekeeper role of the GP. However, this is not considered 'normal' practice.

Traditionally GP services are very broad. GPs are trained more broadly than even American family practitioners. Personal, first-contact care includes diagnostic assessment and management of presenting symptoms/problems, and follow up if necessary. Registration encourages long-term and continuing care of families, as well as individuals, so that physician and patient get to know each other over years of contact. The GP works in a relatively stable community with a population base of approximately 2,000. The content of work (morbidity) is what can be expected in a population denominator of this size, namely a predominance of minor and chronic disorders and low prevalence of dramatic life-threatening situations.

In addition, the GP is well placed, together with colleagues in the primary-care team, to take on responsibilities for community care, seeking out at-risk groups and promoting health and preventing problems. In fact the GP is in a position to act as a controller for the rest of specialist and other services, coordinating and facilitating them for the benefit of his or her patients.

In the UK, changes in the NHS mean that a greater proportion of care will be provided outside hospitals, by general practitioners and associated community health services. One development is a shift towards 'shared care'. In shared care schemes, GPs, practice teams and community health staff are involved in routine management and monitoring activities that have formerly been the province of hospital doctors. Shared care with local specialists, along agreed guidelines, exists for patients with asthma, diabetes, cancer and other groups and this may often involve specialists visiting the practices to consult. The work of general practice involves office consultations and clinics, home visits, care of those in nursing homes and visits to patients in hospital (but with no hospital privileges). All these services are at no cost to patients, they are all part of the NHS general practice.

For example:

- patients discharged from hospital will be visited by nurses from the practice at home

- disabled patients will receive daily visits for care, baths by nurses, etc.

- mothers with new babies will be visited by community midwives and later health visitors at home.

The 1990 contract for GPs now links their income and extra fees to public policies for prevention and health promotion. These extra fees include meeting targets for achieving immunization of over 90% of children registered with the GP and reaching targets for pap smears in 80% of women aged between 20 and 65; for checkups of new patients; for running health promotion programmes in the practice; and for examining regularly all persons aged over 75.

There is almost no private general practice in the UK, apart from a very few completely private practices in parts of London. The private insurance medical schemes do not cover general practice; rather, they provide supplementary coverage, largely of elective surgery, and other procedures, that allow policy holders to by-pass waiting lists and be seen promptly.

There is no two-tier system of quality in British general practice or specialty care. The overall quality of British clinicians is recognized throughout Europe. Specialists are trained longer than in the US, and under the direct supervision of senior mentors.

Public hospitals, analogous to Belview Hospital in New York, have long been the major centers of excellence. Private hospitals have been relatively uncommon and more superficially equipped. Standards are assessed through regular checks and visits to practice premises, and by annual reports.

With the increasing role of management in General Practice quality assurance is being implemented. Currently many FHSAs carry out an annual practice visit to assess standards and criteria in both the clinical and non-clinical areas. Each year a practice is required to submit an annual report to the FHSA which forms part of the monitoring process.

Comprehensive Care and Finance

The extent of primary care services in the British NHS is extensive. It extends well beyond traditional, medical care by physicians; from genetic counselling to minor surgery, from pregnancy and delivery to geriatrics and care of the dying.

Table 3.3 NHS sources of funds and expenditures (OHE, 1992)

Sources of funds	Proportion (percentage)
• general taxes	80
• specific national health insurance	15
• other sources	5
Expenditure	
• hospital services	60
general medical services (general practice) (including prescribed drugs)	20
• public and community preventive and health promotional services	20

(NHS administrative costs are 11%)

Table 3.4 NHS workforce and medical manpower. The NHS is the UK's largest employer involving 1 in 10 of the working population and represents 1 million people. This is made up of the groups below: all groups have increased over the last 40 years and particularly administrators, physicians and technicians

	1992	Ratio 1951–1992
Physicians	10%	× 3.5
Nurses	50%	× 2.2
Administrators	20%	× 5.6
Technicians	15%	× 6.8
Others	5%	× 0.8

Within the primary-care team ideology the GP works with practice nurses, home nurses, community psychiatric workers, counselors, public health nurses (home visitors) and community midwives. Under the new fundholding scheme the practices can, and many do, employ or contract physiotherapists, chiropractors, podiatrists (chiropodists) and complementary (alternative) medicine practitioners. The larger GP practices may also contract for specialty and hospital services, putting them in the seat of power over most medical services. The work of the practice team extends to the community and working with social workers 'at risk' groups are defined and targeted for special care and services.

The NHS is largely funded from public taxation and more than half the expenditure is on hospital services with 20% on general practice. Over the last 40 years the proportion of government expenditure on health has increased from 12% in 1950 to 15% in 1991 (Table 3.3).

There are approximately 100,000 physicians (1 to 575 population); the figure can be broken down and explained as follows (Table 3.4):

- the 20,000 hospital specialists or 'consultants', who are physicians appointed to senior NHS appointments

- 40,000 'junior hospital doctors', who are in training positions from interns to residents and to registrars – these training appointments may be from 6 to 15 years depending on the specialty, and some will include future GPs

- 33,500 'GP principals' – those who have completed a 5-year training, including a 3 year mandatory vocational training scheme, and who have been accepted by FHSAs as principals allowed to accept 'registered patients'

- 2,100 'vocational trainees' who work in approved GP training practices for 1 year at the end of their 3-year period and then seek to become principals

- 500 'assistants' or 'associates', who are salaried part-timers employed by some practices

- 7,000 others, including physicians working in public and community health services, administration and related appointments.

Each District General Hospital (DGH) serves 250,000 people and employs 4,250 staff, of the staff, doctors represent 5% with nurses and midwives 53%.

Training periods after medical school for specialists in the UK, until they are appointed as 'consultants' (recognized NHS specialists) are much longer than for GP principals (Table 3.5).

Following the 5–6 years of undergraduate medical training, after graduating from an academic high school track, there is a 1-year pre-registration period before being registered as a medical practitioner, and for general practice a

Table 3.5 Training periods for UK physicians

General practitioners		Specialists	
Pre-registration (intern)	1 year	Pre-registration/ Senior House Officer (intern/resident)	3 years
Vocational training (trainee-resident)	3 years	Registrar (senior resident)	4 years
Possibly extra	1–2 years	Senior Registrar (Fellow/Assistant Professor)	4 years
Total	5–6 years	Total	11 years

further mandatory 3-year vocational training program (2 years hospital and 1 year general practice) (Chapter 6).

The mandatory vocational training program for GPs is 3 years; 1.5–2 years spent in hospital posts, and 1–1.5 years in an approved, training general practice. There are 2,500 training practices in the UK and around 2,000 trainees. The scheme is financed by the NHS and organized and administered from national to local levels. GP trainers and practices are carefully selected and supervized. Trainees have to be approved at the end of their training and are encouraged to take the membership examination of the RCGP. The approval of trainees is moving from a formative to a summative assessment from January 1996.

With a national health system it is possible to have national manpower policies. Since medical education is tuition free to the students, and since about four out of five of all graduates will work for the NHS, long-term planning controls are possible. There are committees that recommend numbers of medical students, numbers of physicians likely to be needed for general practice and other specialties and numbers in training posts.

There is control of the distribution of GPs and this has resulted in an equable distribution of physicians. There are no areas of shortages of GPs in the UK, but surpluses (based on population per GP) in one fifth of the UK. The average list size per NHS GP principal was down to 1,870 in 1991.

The annual growth rate of the total number of physicians in the NHS has been 1.5% over the past 20 years. This means 1,500 extra physicians in the NHS each year in the UK. There are 28 medical schools graduating almost 4,000 new physicians each year, and half of these are women. Training for specialists and GPs is controlled through the General Medical Council (GMC) and the professional colleges.

Physician Income

General Practice

Pay of GPs is negotiated between the medical profession and government through the independent Doctors' and Dentists' Pay Review Body. Annual payments comprise the following:

- capitation fees for each registered patient (extra for over-65s)

- fees for many extra, specified services such as preventive immunization and pap (cervical) smears, minor surgery, medical checks, health promotion clinics, night home visits

- basic practice expenses

- computer grants (63% of practices are computerized)

- reimbursement for use of practice and premises

- reimbursement of 70% of staff wages

- continuing medical education (up to 2,000 per year (3,000))

- additional grants for working in 'deprived areas'

- fees for training young physicians and students if selected as a training practice.

In addition, as a result of recent NHS reforms larger practices (over 7,000 patients) can apply to become fundholders and be given grants of £100 ($150) per patient to purchase hospital services, drug costs and staff salaries. This means that some group practitioners may have annual turnovers of some £2–3 million ($3–5 million). Any savings can be used to improve practice facilities.

Furthermore, NHS GPs are allowed to earn incomes outside the NHS on their own time from insurance work, occupational medicine, as police physicians, writing, lecturing, media appearances, research grants and clinical assistant posts in the hospital.

Income

The annual personal income of GPs (1994) ranged between £100,000 ($150,000) and £35,000 ($52,000) (Table 3.6).

Hospital physicians are paid by salaries, which are also recommended by the Doctors' and Dentists' Pay Review Body (average £52,000 in 1994 ($78,000)) plus 'merit awards' for one third of specialists. NHS specialists receive salary scales depending on seniority and number of weekly, half-day sessions worked. All are paid on the same salary scale. Specialists can also undertake private work out of their hours spent on NHS work. They can and do contract to work seven or even nine of the 11 half-day sessions for the NHS and work privately the rest of the time. Most private work pertains to elective surgery. The average consultant works a sixth of their time in private practice.

The annual income for NHS specialists is shown in Table 3.7.

The total of £102,000 ($150,000) is approximate and incomes of some specialists may be much higher from merit awards and private fees. Note that the

Table 3.6 Average annual income for GPs

NHS recommended taxable income	£42,000 ($63,000)
Expenses (NHS) (added to income to pay for equipment etc.)	£22,500 ($33,750)
Non-NHS fees	£10,000 ($15,000)
Total	£74,500 ($111,750)

Table 3.7 Average annual income for specialists

NHS recommended salary	£52,000 ($78,000)
Possible merit award (average)	£20,000 ($30,000)
Private practice (wide range)	£30,000 ($45,000)
Total	£102,000 ($153,000)

basic differential rates of pay for the NHS GP and NHS specialist is 1:1.25, which is much less than in the US.

Reorganization

1991–1993

During its 45 years (1948–1993) the NHS has undergone periodic changes in policies and directions from the political parties in power, most recently in 1990–1993. In 1987, the Conservative Government was subjected to considerable public criticism of the NHS over delays in care, shortages of resources and lack of funding. In response the Prime Minister, Margaret Thatcher, set up her own secret review of the NHS, with a promise to report to the nation within a year. This she did in a White Paper (of recommendations to Parliament) titled *Working For Patients* (1989). The 'diagnosis' of the Prime Minister's committee was not shortage of funding but of managerial inefficiencies and lack of competition. The 'remedies' proposed were structural without any changes to the basic NHS concepts of funding from general taxation and free care at point of service and no one priced out or denied any care on account of high costs of treatment (*see also* Chapter 6).

To summarize points made in *Working for Patients*:

- competitive internal market with managed care within the NHS (but little 'privatization')
- providing and purchasing services at competitive prices
- firm contracts to be made, carried out and monitored
- accountability.

Hospitals and other health facilities are to be encouraged to become independent provider units as trusts. General practitioners to become fundholders with generous funds to purchase competitively, for their patients' elective, specialty care (emergency and high cost services excluded) and admissions as well as the staff costs, prescribing costs, tests, overheads, data collection and analysis and various other services of the GP practice.

Physicians' incomes were not included and were paid normally. Money saved could be used to improve the practice but could not be kept personally. The annual GP budgets were approximately £100 ($150) per registered citizen plus extra allowances for developing the scheme.

1994 Onwards

Further changes in the NHS are taking place with the abolition of Regional Health Authorities and the merger of District Health Authorities and FHSAs from April 1996.

There will also be a new and more effective management chain from the center to the periphery – with new NHS Policy Board and NHS Management Executive at the DoH and relating to local management structures at regional and district levels and with FHSAs.

These proposed changes are expected to:

- improve data collection through national, synchronized, computerized collection to include audits in hospitals and general practice

- provide more management accountability of physicians and some checks of complete clinical freedom

- reduce NHS management with the release of more money for direct patient care

- decentralize the NHS with regional and district planning of resources relating to the needs of the local population

- clarify role and responsibilities

- provide cost-effective health care.

The Patient's Charter

In 1992 the DoH produced outlines for a Patient's Charter to increase accountability and consumer pressure. This provided guidelines and standards for users and providers, rather than rigid directives.

From April 1993, GP practices were asked to produce quality standards to include: maximum waiting times for appointments, arrangements for receiving and passing messages, response to emergencies and requests for home visits, the needs of minority groups, disease prevention and health promotion. This is in addition to annual health reports and information leaflets on practice organization and arrangements. Many practices are also setting out what they see as the patients' own responsibilities in the form of 'Practice Charters'.

After a period of bitter dissent between the Government, the political opposition, professional organizations, the media and the public, it was remarkable that the new Act of Parliament was passed in April 1991. Even more remarkably its implementation has been more smooth than expected and without major disruptions to health care services. It has not yet been possible to evaluate the successes and failures – we must await reliable independent data.

What can be said is that the NHS percentage of GDP funding has increased little, priority decisions (rationing) still exist and management changes have created much stress and disharmony. But patients continue to receive appropriate care albeit with occasional difficulties and problems from the changes.

In the future the role of primary care is likely to increase further, based on locality management and patient needs. We will see the development of new approaches to managing primary care, the relating of practice activity to local needs, development of additional services and an increased understanding of closer networks between smaller practices.

Initially primary care teams will be developed with an improved measurement of health gain of many aspects of patient management. As these changes occur shared care between primary and secondary care will become established, driven by fundholding practices.

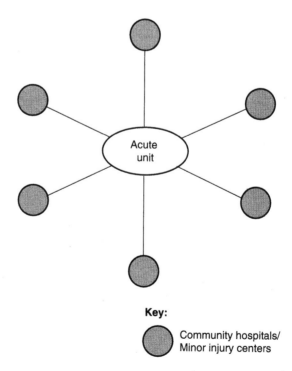

Figure 3.1 The Future of Secondary Care.

Following on from this, community hospital and respite care will expand and it is likely that the future model of secondary care will involve a central acute provider unit supported by a number of community hospitals and minor injury centers etc. Community targets will become established (Figure 3.1).

Summary

After 45 years, the NHS is an essential part of the British social fabric. It is popular with the people and the professionals and has passed through a series of administrative reorganization, but its basic structure is the same. It provides free care at the time of service, of generally sound and equal quality and is a single tier system. There is a complementary private medical insurance scheme, it covers only 11% of the population, is for elective specialist services only and is voluntary. The scheme tends to be associated with employment perks, and deals chiefly with elective surgical procedures. It is generally accepted that the facilities for major medical problems are much more comprehensive in the NHS!

No national health system is perfect – nor is the NHS. It is endeavoring to cope with resources that do not meet all needs and wants, leading to waits and delays in some areas, such as cold surgical procedures, but acute and major problems are managed without due delays.

In the future, managed care will be developed further on a locality basis and primary care's role will expand. The hospital will change with the development of community units and a central acute unit on a locality basis. The National Health Service will provide a basic package of health care with additional services provided by alternative funding. Rationing of health care will become inevitable.

4

The US Health Care System

Introduction

The US is a young nation born out of pioneers and with philosophies of equality of opportunities, freedom and democracy, self-reliance and entrepreneurship – all of which have been transmitted into the health care system.

There is no single system; health care is provided through a multi-mix of private and public schemes. Private insurance through employment covers most of the population, but it is not full and comprehensive. Publicly funded programs like Medicare (for the elderly), Medicaid (for the poor) and state schemes have slowly filled the gaps over the decades and now generate over 40% of health costs. Personal out-of-pocket payments are the highest of developed countries and make up almost one third of patient expenses, although there are some special, voluntary and charitable programs to help the poor or those without insurance through work, but a sizeable proportion of the population (17%) has no medical insurance.

The US health system is the most expensive at over 14% of GDP, or $3,600 per head in 1993, and may reach 15% of GDP or $5,000 per head, by the year 2000. There is no shortage of physicians and the rate per population is higher than in many other countries. Nor does there appear to be a dearth of primary physicians, but they are distributed unevenly and have poorly defined roles.

While there are recognizable levels of professional care the lines are blurred because of the patient's free choice and access to any physician, the lack of gatekeeping roles for primary physicians, and the mixture of generalists and specialists. Primary care is in crisis with falling recruitment, uncertainty of roles, and low status. The fragmentation of primary care physicians, with family physicians, general internists and general pediatricians having varying responsibilities, leads to unnecessary competition and a waste of resources.

A priority for the future must be to achieve a national health system more appropriate to the needs of the US people and with primary care playing its part to the full.

The Nation

American policies still reflect the nation's original emphasis on personal freedom and minimal government interference. Such historical factors have been translated into features of its health system and services, largely through the efforts of the medical profession. Thus professional autonomy, free choice and treating citizens as self-reliant individuals until they come in for help, have characterized the US health care system. Private individual charges, voluntary insurance and public support only for the needy and elderly, have been the financial principles underlying the system. Although it is the funding mechanisms and levels that have impeded equal access to services, most Americans believe that governmental programs are inefficient and unresponsive. It has often been noted that the US and South Africa are the only industrialized countries without universal health insurance or a national health system.

The US is a vast, diverse and changing society. About one million new immigrants enter each year, half of them illegally. Its multi-ethnic groups are growing more numerous and more distinct. At present, caucasians of many origins make up 75%, African-Americans 12%, and Hispanics, Asians and others 13% of the population. It is these last groups that are the majority of the new immigrants. More than one in five of the population is under 15 years, but the society is aging fast (13% over 65) because of falling birth rates and longer life (Table 4.1).

Health indices overall are among the lowest of industrialized nations and vary dramatically by educational, income and ethnic group. Paradoxically, this affluent and successful nation is afflicted with many modern social pathologies in its rates of crime, homicide, drug abuse, AIDS and poverty, which are substantially higher than in other nations.

With varied health needs, mainly not addressed by the existing health care system, and spiraling medical expenses that exceed 14% of GDP, the nation seeks a new delivery system that can guarantee access for all yet hold costs down.

Origins of the Health Care System

The modern American health care system arose from a wide range of therapies practiced by large numbers of healers in the late 19th century. This frustrated the American Medical Association (AMA) and its leaders trained in the new scientific medicine. Through a series of remarkably successful campaigns, the AMA and state medical societies gained control of medical education and licensure on behalf of scientific medicine. The systematic improvement in medical education at the beginning of the century was followed by the increasing importance of the hospital, the specialization of most physicians and the rise of the research oriented academic medical center in the mid-century.

Table 4.1 Demography (US:UK) (*The Economist*, 1992; Health US, 1990; National Center for Health Statistics, 1991; OHE, 1992)

	UK	US
Population (millions)	57.5	250
(annual growth)	(0.3%)	(1%)
Population		
Under 15	18.9%	21.4%
Over 65	15.5%	12.6%
Birth rate		
Annual per 1,000 population	13.4	14.1
Cesarean section rate per births	10%	25%
Infant mortality per 1,000 births	8.4	9.0
Legal abortions		
per 1,000 women	11.7	28.0
per 100 births	18.0	29.7
Fertility rate		
(children per woman 15–45)	1.8	1.9
Life expectancy (at birth)	M 72	M 73
	F 78	F 80
Deaths		
Annual per 1,000	11.4	8.3
Place of death (hospital)	65%	75%
Social		
Unemployed workers	9%	8%
Marriage (annual per 1,000 population)	6.7	9.7
Divorce (annual per 1,000 population)	2.9	4.8
Number persons per household	2.6	2.8
Wealth		
Annual GDP per capita ($)	16.000	21.700
Health expenditure		
% GDP	6.3	12 +
(Public)	(5.3)	(4.8)
(Private)	(1.0)	(7.2)

The shift in the locus of care and a mounting pile of unpaid bills caused by the Depression led hospitals and then doctors to create provider-run, non-profit health insurance on a voluntary basis. Commercial insurers joined in, and coverage rapidly expanded, providing pass-through reimbursement for hospital and specialty care. The proportion of physicians who were general practitioners (GPs) fell from 75% in 1935, to 45% in 1957, to 34% in 1990.

Between the 1930s and the 1980s the AMA, along with other provider groups successfully opposed national health insurance and emphasized employer-based insurance that paid for care only when billed by physicians and hospitals (Starr, 1982). Thus most medicine was done by private practitioners, clinics and hospitals who charged fees.

When Congress finally legislated in 1965 coverage for the elderly (Medicare) and the poor (Medicaid), it reinforced the fee for service payments. Direct federal funds were confined largely to capital for building more hospital beds and for research. Thus by the late 1960s, the majority of doctors were specialists, there developed a crisis in primary care, and costs began to rise rapidly. People could see any specialists they wished – and did. Few physicians chose to go into general practice and those few were isolated from the mainstream medical community. Hospitals expanded rapidly and competed to offer the latest in technical services, which were generously reimbursed. The term 'medical-industrial complex' appeared, and the protected markets of medical services flourished at high profits.

The Structure

From this brief history one can see that the organization of the American system is a loose one, emphasizing the hospital and technical services. There is a blurring between all four levels of care (*see* Chapter 2), because there is no clear division of labor between generalists and specialists. An arrangement to this end was discussed earlier this century but rejected because GPs wanted to retain hospital privileges (Stevens, 1971).

General Practice Among Specialists

Since the 1960s, the primary care vacuum has meant in effect that much 'primary care' is done by specialists, what Fry (1960) called 'specialoids' (*see also* p. 60). To fill the vacuum, internal medicine, pediatrics, obstetrics, and psychiatry each declared themselves to be a 'primary care specialty', and all but psychiatry have succeeded. In fact, about 80% of internists and 50% of pediatricians end up in subspecialties, but all American statistics count them as primary care doctors.

Most important, after years of campaigning, general practice attained specialty status by requiring residency training and board certification centered on its new focus, family practice. The Millis Report of 1966 proposed that primary care be recognized as a specialty and receive federal funding and that community health centers be established in poor areas. Both of these changes were made, and the American Board of Family Practice was established in 1969. This change partially stopped the loss of physicians in primary care by encouraging

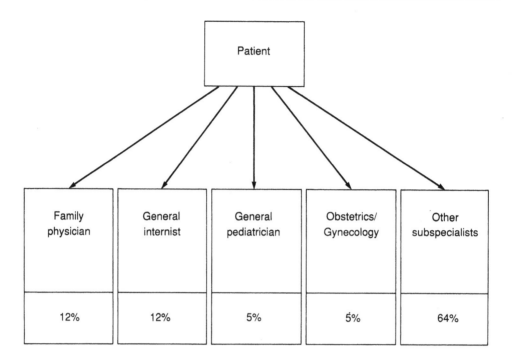

Figure 4.1 Per cent Distribution of US Generalist and Specialty Physicians.

thousands of new doctors to become residency trained. However, as older GPs retire, there has continued to be a significant decrease in the percentage of American physicians in general and family practice.

Family physicians (FPs) and general internists represent the largest groups to whom people turn for primary care. They provide a wide range of services, but a different blend from the British GPs who have access to a broader range of resources through the NHS. Patients go to a wide variety of generalists and specialists for first-contact care, as illustrated in Figure 4.1. With some exceptions, there is no counterpart to community nursing, primary medical teams, and the wide array of services for the disabled, the chronically ill, and the feeble. Home health care is expanding in the US, but largely as a set of high-tech services (such as home intravenous therapy or home physical therapy) provided by for-profit teams. US FPs and internists take care of hospitalized patients and do more procedures (such as sigmoidoscopy) than British GPs.

About 39% of all expenditures go on hospital services, and this percentage has been dropping slightly as insurers and government programs have become much more strict about hospital admissions and length of stay. American hospital lengths of stay are the shortest in the world, but also the most expensive, because those few days are packed with sophisticated procedures, advanced equipment, and highly trained staff working in expensively built facilities. As more and more complex procedures are done on an out-patient basis, doctors and hospitals have been competing for market share. Many have joined forces to establish surgi-centers, women's centers, imaging centers etc., so that the term 'hospital' now includes many facilities and side corporations besides the central building with in-patient beds. Recently there has also been a strong trend to 'vertical integration', with hospitals setting up organizations to be involved in and potentially control all aspects of patient care from primary-care practice to nursing homes.

Medical Manpower

Surprisingly, the manpower crisis of the late 1960s precipitated a major federal program to expand medical schools. In fact, much of the 'crisis' stemmed from there being too few generalists and too many specialists. The number of graduates doubled, and the number of doctors has been expanding rapidly ever since. However, in the absence of an overall manpower plan, most graduates have chosen specialty training. By the mid-1970s, a surplus was predicted in all but a few of the specialties.

From 1965 to 1990, the numbers of family practitioners in the US declined slowly (0.1% per annum), while general internists and general pediatricians rose by 6% annually. Specialists rose much faster so that the percentage of primary care doctors fell from 43 in 1965 to 34 in 1990 (Table 4.2).

Many of the new physicians are women, and they now make up 40–60% of medical school classes. Intensive recruitment of minorities has generated only a slowly increasing number of candidates against the many other careers open to the talented. What used to be called 'foreign medical graduates' (FMGs) became a significant factor in the 1960s, when rapidly expanding hospital and specialty programs searched for young doctors, who had graduated from non-US medical schools, to fill the more unpopular (inner city) residencies. After medical schools doubled the national class size, there was increasing pressure to cut back on FMGs. An increasing number of them, however, were Americans who went abroad to obtain a medical degree, and their families mounted a powerful lobby. Subsequent actions have neutralized the term to 'international medical graduates' (IMGs) and tightened standards, slowly reducing their proportion from 32% of residents in 1970 to 23% in 1990. IMGs tend to fill empty residency slots, many of them now in internal medicine.

Financing Medical Care

The voluntary health insurance system works best in mid-size and large companies, which provide coverage for employees and their dependents as a benefit.

Table 4.2 Proliferation of provider

Practitioners	1960	1980	2000
Physicians (MDs, DOs)	251,200	457,500	704,700
Persons per active physician	735	508	369
Chiropractors	unknown	24,400	88,100
Registered nurses[a]	592,000	1,272,900	1,900,000
Licensed practical nurses[a]	217,000	549,300	724,500
Nurse-midwives[b]	500(?)	2,000	4,800
Physician assistants[c]	0	11,000	32,800
Nurse-practitioners[d]	0	14,700	36,400

[a] The figure for 2,000 was an interpolation between high and low estimates.
[b] The figure for 2,000 was calculated by assuming 200 graduates per year, with gross attrition rate of 20%.
[c] The figure for 1980 was based on the figure for 1983 minus attrition projected back to 1980; the figure for 2,000 was calculated by assuming 1,500 graduates per year, with gross attrition rate of 20%.
[d] The figure for 2,000 was calculated by assuming 2,100 graduates per year, with gross attrition rate of 20%.

Employers typically pay a 'middle-man' insurance company, who then administers the benefits and pays the doctors and hospitals. Some employers offer employees a range of insurance policies to choose from, each administered by a different company. Each policy may cover different services, have different charges and co-payments to the employee and involve different doctors and hospitals. Some companies are 'self-insured' and administer the plan themselves or contract with only one insurance company to do so. These policies are 'experience-rated', which means that the premiums reflect the health status and illnesses of each employee group. As firm size falls below 50 employees, so the percentage of companies providing health insurance drops rapidly, and staff in these companies must buy insurance on an individual basis (which is very expensive – often double or triple the cost to the employer) or through volunteer associations to which they belong (these plans are uncommon and usually involve very large deductibles and co-insurance).

Many large companies also cover employees' dependents, often for an additional charge. Because of the wide variability of medical coverage by employers and the universal exclusion of coverage for pre-existing conditions in new employees, many people are reluctant to change jobs and run the risk of receiving markedly fewer, or no benefits.

Another complicating factor in the American medical care system is that companies are usually searching for a cheaper health plan; they may change the types and numbers of plans offered to employees annually (who may shift plans once a year). Each plan may contract with only a certain number of physicians or hospitals, so that long-term continuity of care is impossible. Both patients and physicians are confused as to what is actually covered and what has been carried out before by other clinicians or facilities. Insurance plans adopt a one-year mentality, in part because employees are likely to change plans, and in part to make a profit by minimizing the amount of medical or hospital bills paid for that year. Thus they are unlikely to invest in preventive care, and they put as many administrative hurdles as possible in the way of getting care (Light, 1993).

Medicare was provided for the elderly, when a plan focused on hospital and specialty care; ironically it covers few home or long-term services for the chronically ill. In addition, Medicare often covers only a portion of physician bills, no drug costs, no other health professions (such as dentists or psychologists), and has significant deductibles before any charges are paid. Because of these gaps in coverage, over 80% of the elderly purchase a supplementary insurance policy for relatively high premiums to help with the uncovered expenses.

Under federal law, the states also provide Medicaid for the poor, with the Federal Government paying about half the costs, more for poorer states and less for affluent ones. The 50 states, however, have made very different decisions about how many services they will cover and about who is eligible. On the whole, they use strict eligibility rules that allow only half or less of those with survival incomes (the poverty line) to be covered – primarily poor women with children and poor elderly with chronic disorders who have used up all their life savings paying for what Medicare does not cover. Once their savings are below about $2,000, they become eligible for Medicaid, which does pay for long-term care and a broad range of home services as well as all acute services. In some states, only a third of those on survival incomes are eligible.

Another difficulty is that payment levels for most Medicaid services are set so low that only a few providers will treat Medicaid patients. These providers may 'compensate' by treating a high volume of poor patients.

For many years, about 35 million Americans have had no health insurance. Three quarters of these uninsured are in working families. Latinos and African-Americans are twice as likely to be uninsured. When they need care, these citizens (one in every six) use the relatively small and underfunded system of public hospital emergency rooms and clinics, as well as non-physician providers and healers.

An unknown but estimated 40 to 70 million Americans have 'Swiss cheese policies' with substantial holes of medical insurance coverage in the middle (exclusion clauses for not covering existing illnesses or high risks, ranging from mental illness to pregnancy, to diabetes), on the front edge (increased deductibles), the sides (co-payments), or the back edge (payment caps). No systematic records are kept of these internal policy features, but they have perpetrated a crisis for both physicians and their patients (Light, 1992a). There are over 1200 insurance companies selling medical insurance. Because they compete on price, and because there is no definition of what must be covered by insurance, almost every conceivable and confusing exclusion is used to reduce claims paid.

To illustrate how such policies work, a patient must first pay the annual deductible ($300–800) and then the co-payment (20–50%) on 'reasonable' or 'allowable' charges. These charge levels are increasingly set well below typical levels of billing. Thus a patient with a $1,200 bill for diagnostic tests and fees might first pay the yearly deductible (say, $400) and then 20% of the allowable charge, *plus* the remainder of the bill. If the insurer allowed $800 as a 'reasonable' or 'allowable' charge, it would pay $320 (80% of $400) and the patient would pay $880 ($400 deductible + $80 for 20% of the allowable charge + $400 for the remainder of the bill). In this common case, the patient would pay 73.3% out of pocket. For the second such bill, the patient would not pay the deductible, reducing out-of-pocket costs to 40% (Light, 1992). However, each year the deductible must be paid out of pocket before the medical insurance plan pays anything.

Since the mid-1970s, employers have initiated a number of changes to restrain rising costs:

- health insurance benefits that cover more of bills if patients choose providers in the plan under contract to charge less

- increases in deductibles, partial payments by patients (co-payments), or co-premiums

- volume discount contracts to selected groups of providers called PPOs (Preferred Provider Organizations)

- utilization review by the insurance company to prevent unnecessary procedures and reduce hospital days.

This effort has greatly expanded forms of managed care but has not slowed medical expenses, though many large companies feel their plan has lowered their rate of premium increases. It has, however, shifted costs back to employees, particularly those employees belonging to plans less aggressive about cost containment. Cost saving has turned out to be largely buck-passing.

Overall, the voluntary competitive insurance system lies at the root of a number of problems, we believe, for both patients and doctors, as shown below.

1. Lack of standardization of medical plans; so many variations that neither doctors nor patients can determine in advance how much of a full treatment plan will be covered.

2. Millions spent by insurance companies to figure out how *not* to enroll potentially high utilizing patients, how not to cover people when they are sick and most need coverage, or *not* pay covered bills when they come in.

3. Use of experience or risk rating by group, greatly increasing premiums for small groups and individuals, many of whom decide not to have insurance.

4. Laws (especially ERISA)* make it nearly impossible for states to ensure that patients are covered fairly and that allow self-insured companies to circumvent state laws on health insurance.

5. Barriers to changing jobs; one in three Americans said they would change jobs were it not for the fear of losing insurance coverage for medical services.

6. Profit motive spurring employers and insurers to the activities in (2) and to switch plans on employees to avoid paying for costly illnesses, within a short-term, year-to-year framework.

7. Huge administrative costs, estimated to be as high as 25% of all health care expenditures (Woolhandler and Himmelstein, 1991). For example, we estimate there are five billion claims a year just for office visits to doctors; immense paper work for the provider (up to 100 billing staff for a 300-bed hospital), for the patient, and for the insurance company (up to 100 claims payment staff per 100,000 enrollees).

The US health care financing system is now like a giant shell game, every payer trying to shift costs to other payers, especially back to the patient or to the doctor in the form of unpaid or partially paid bills. In addition, patients pay 30% of all medical costs out of their own pockets. When insurance companies or patients do not pay part or all of a claim, the providers often come after patients through collection agencies, which have the power of ruining their credit for all other financing in their lives.

These problems have led to widespread dissatisfaction of both patients and physicians. The US spends the most money on health care yet registers the highest consumer dissatisfaction with their medical care of any industrialized nation (Blendon and Edwards, 1991).

---

*Employee Retirement Income Security Act (1974) which prohibits states from regulating self-insured employee health plans. Only the Federal Government can, and so far has chosen not to do so.

Physician Income

Although physician costs are about 20% of total medical costs and half of that goes to overhead expenses, only 10% of all health care dollars go to physicians' 'take-home' pay. However, this still amounts to very high incomes; among the highest in the world. Most doctors still bill privately and are paid on a fee-for-service basis. But a growing number work for a salary plus bonuses, for a contract, or on the basis of capitation fees in various managed care organizations. This situation is complex and changing rapidly.

Primary care doctors and a few specialties that involve considerable listening or counselling (such as psychiatry and geriatrics) average about $100,000 per year. Many of the medical subspecialties, such as cardiology, gastroenterology, general surgery and obstetrics and gynecology, average about $200,000, while subspecialty surgeons, such as orthopedics, cardiothoracic and neurosurgery, average over $300,000 (AAFP, 1992 and Light, 1993). These are 1990 figures, and although the mean is about 150,000, there is a long right-handed tail to the distribution stretching out to 800,000 or more. These payment patterns date back to the payments committees of Blue Cross and other insurance plans, which were dominated by hospital-based specialties. They reflect higher charges allowed for new 'experimental' procedures, the use of which soon becomes widespread (such as laparoscopy), and also reflect critical moments when, for example, radiologists and pathologists refused to be billed as part of hospital services and set up independent businesses that contract with several hospitals. The so-called competition of the last 15 years has generally not brought down the earnings of these high-end specialties. Indeed, this disparity has been exaggerated. In the 1960s, specialists typically earned 50% more than primary care physicians; now, it is two to three times as much. These dramatic inequities in earnings, without any difference in hours worked (about 55 per week) are one of the key reasons for students deciding to pursue subspecialty careers.

Organization of Services

From 1970 to the late 1980s, there was a steady trend of less hospitalization and a shift back to office-based care for patients. Most doctors (82%) are principally involved in patient care (the remainder in teaching, research or administration), and despite all the talk today about physician-executives, the data show no notable increase (Roback, Randolph and Seidman, 1990: Table A-2). The number of physicians in office-based practice (not associated with a hospital) has been rising slowly since 1970 (from 55% to 58.5%), and the percentage of physicians practicing full-time in hospitals has declined from 10.4 to 8.5. However, hospital-based practice makes up 23.6% of all practice sites because of all the residents and fellows in training. This underscores the immense role that medical education, as practically an industry in itself, plays in manning and supporting hospital-based practice. The total number of residents has grown since 1970 by 60%, and they are a major source of 'cheap' labor.

An increasing number of the 58% of doctors practicing in 'offices' (ie not a hospital or institution) do so in groups. Since the mid-1960s, when private and public insurance became fully established and funded expansion with few restraints, more and more doctors have combined into groups to form professional corporations.

While there were 4,300 groups in 1965, this figure rose to 8,500 in 1975 and 16,600 in 1988 (Havlicek, 1990: Chapter 8). This means that while 11% of all non-federal physicians worked in group practice in 1965, 30% did so by 1988. Supporting this emphasis on economic rather than service motives, an increasing percentage practise in single specialty groups, up from 54% in 1975 to 71% in 1988. These groups tend to be small, with an average of 6.2 physicians in 1988, and their purpose is largely to share the financing of space, staff and equipment, and to position themselves for handling larger contracts from institutional payers.

An important, perhaps even integral part of the rapid expansion of groups since the mid-1970s has involved doctors investing in their own clinical laboratories, radiology labs, electro-cardiological labs and audiology labs. (In addition, 40% of all office-based physicians have their own labs for blood tests or sample cultures.) The larger the group, the more likely it will own one or more of these facilities.

For example, while 23% of three-person groups own clinical labs, this rises steadily to 78% for groups with more than 75 doctors. Large groups also own their own surgical duties, from 15% of groups size 16–25, to 41% of groups size 76–99. The reason is primarily economic, as current reimbursement levels allow large profits to be made in lab, X-ray and surgical areas. Because the purchase of equipment and staff is so expensive, larger groups are more easily able to afford the initial costs and refer enough patients to keep the facilities busy.

Reorganization Towards Managed Care

In 1970–71, President Richard Nixon, Senator Edward Kennedy (who chaired the Senate Labor and Human Resources Committee), and the business community (which paid and pays most premiums as an employee benefit) all declared that the health care system was in crisis. Problems included:

- weak and dwindling primary care
- too much surgery, hospital care, tests, and specialty visits

- escalating costs that would soon bankrupt the nation

- fragmented, impersonal care

- millions of uninsured citizens, including half the poor who should have been covered by Medicaid.

Each group proposed its own version of national health insurance and met with opposition by doctors, insurance companies and medical supply companies. However, Nixon's proposal for managed competition between hundreds of health maintenance organizations (HMOs) passed into legislation. HMOs provide nearly all medical services for a fixed subscription per annum. One of the key components of the HMO legislation was that all employers with over 25 employees, who offered medical insurance as a benefit (many do not), must offer an HMO as an option if one exists in the nearby region. Overnight, HMOs had a built-in market.

Currently, managed care in the US means essentially that someone in addition to the physician is trying to decrease medical costs by 'managing' the patient's care through aggressive contracting or utilization controls (Table 4.3). Typically the primary care physician is the key player and could be rewarded by ordering fewer tests or procedures, ie, rewarded for more 'appropriate' utilization.

Table 4.3 Definitions of managed care

Managed care	Any system of health service payment or delivery arrangements where the health plan attempts to control or coordinate use of health services by its enrolled members in order to contain health expenditures, by either improving quality or lowering it
Managed competition	An approach to health system reform in which health plans compete to provide health insurance coverage and services for enrollees. Typically, enrollees sign up with a health plan purchasing entity and choose a service plan during an open enrolment period
Managed indemnity	This is traditional private fee for service care with utilization controls and reimbursement of fees by the insurance company

Managed care now comes in many variants, but a useful framework is provided by the four basic types of HMOs and PPOs.

1. *Staff or group model HMOs* – center around a full-time staff who take care of a defined number of patients (or enrollees). They look like more traditional medical multispecialty groups but with greater numbers of primary care physicians. The groups must figure out how to best serve their subscribers on a fixed budget. These groups are better at holding costs down, primarily by reducing hospital admissions. In staff model HMOs, the plan employs the physicians, while in group models, the plan contracts with medical groups who only take care of that plan's patients.

2. *IPA (Independent Practice Association) HMOs* – contract with hundreds of private physicians, each of whom takes on varying numbers of their subscribers in return for a capitation or fee-for-service contract, plus incentives for holding down hospital and specialty costs. Hundreds of new for-profit HMOs have chosen the IPA approach to increase subscribers' choices and therefore market appeal. Typically, lower start-up costs are needed as physicians still have their own offices and staff. But IPA controls over actual practice patterns are tenuous, which often leads to micromanagement by the IPA central staff or the insurance company to control patient utilization.

3. *Network HMOs* – lie inbetween, contracting with many group practices. This means that some of the clinical management can be done within the groups of colleagues, rather than externally by monitors from the central office. Network HMOs try to combine the best of both worlds – colleague self-management and wide choice for market appeal.

4. *Preferred Provider Organizations (PPOs)* – groups of doctors who offer volume discounts to insurers or employers in return for preferred status (usually by having their reduced fees covered by the subscriber's insurance policy instead of a patient's co-payment). They can be narrow (an obstetrical PPO) or broad (a primary care PPO). Initially hailed as a panacea, they are not proving to save money, and the decrease in fees has been accompanied by an increase in patient volume. PPOs typically do not have a central office to do utilization review; it is more frequently done by the insurance company.

New hybrids have been created to attract more subscribers, such as the Point of Service HMO that allows subscribers to go outside the HMO when they want to see another physician who is not a member of the plan. In that case, the patient ends up paying much more (but not all) of that physician's bill.

Currently, over 50 million Americans get their care from HMOs. This is growing steadily, though much more slowly than envisioned originally. Details of enrollment and disenrollment led some to believe this shows that most

Americans have 'rejected' the restrictions of HMOs and lead others to believe that Americans are being converted. Managed care in less rigorous forms is part of most health insurance plans. Indeed, in many states Medicaid and Medicare are turning to HMOs to enroll their patients. True endemnity medical insurance, where a portion or all of the physician's fee for each service is paid without a contract or review, is getting rare and very expensive. In some areas of the US, only 5% of medical insurance is the old-style indemnity insurance.

Comment

The UK and the US have distinctly different health care systems; one based on a strong foundation of primary care through which all other services are co-ordinated, and the other based on a strong tradition of free choice for doctors to specialize and practice how they want. One nation has a manpower plan based on health care needs of its citizens and a global (though too small) budget. The other has no manpower plan and no budget. One guarantees universal access to primary care services and to all other services a person's doctor thinks useful. The other has no such guarantee and encourages those who can pay to seek any services they like. One has rather uniform and high clinical standards with a good deal of monitoring for quality by hand-picked senior specialists. The other has high standards of training but a tradition of autonomy that is paradoxically now leading to micromanagement and loss of physician autonomy. One costs about a third of the other.

Unfortunately, one has to report that the $900 billion paid for medical care in the US in 1993 has bought:

- far more specialists and specialty services than the patterns of illness warrant

- inadequate access, facilities and treatment for the poor and uninsured

- medical impoverishment from uninsured portions of medical bills

- a pluralistic system with multiple types of practice arrangements and payment systems

- a huge, bureaucratic administrative medical insurance system

- lack of public and political agreement on what a future system should look like.

It has also bought:

- modern and well-equipped hospitals and clinics

- high rates of diagnostic tests, treatment, surgery and iatrogenic disorders

- excellent access to many life-saving and disability-reducing procedures for the insured

- an outstanding research establishment.

Conclusion

The US medical system is in the midst of rapid change. Whether or not the Congress passes sweeping legislation to correct the lack of universal coverage, changes will continue. These changes include:

- increasing control by employers of how their medical care dollars are spent

- a weakening of hospitals' control over the organization and financing of medical care

- increasing formation and growth of physician group practices

- increasing managed care (by insurance companies and physicians), with increasing numbers of people taken care of by HMOs and few people insured through plans offering indemnity coverage or contracting with PPOs

- less choice (for patients) of doctors and hospitals.

However, without additional national congressional action, these financing and power changes may slow the acceleration in medical costs, but are unlikely to curtail the growth entirely. They fail to address many issues which are a necessary part of reform, including: malpractice and tort reform, simplification of the administration/financing of the medical system, and an over-reliance on technology to diagnose and treat illness.

Only through addressing the basic building block of any medical system – medical care – can the US make the kind of organizational and philosophical changes that will help the system evolve into one which is more efficient and effective. Primary care physicians are the key to appropriate triage and referrals, to co-ordinated and comprehensive care, and to patient education and community orientation.

5

Primary Care

Introduction

Primary care is an essential level of health care in every health system. It is that level of professional care with which a person or family comes into contact when they decide to seek help. In addition to responsibilities to individuals and families, the primary physician must also accept those of local communities. At this first contact level the content of work mostly comprises common minor and chronic conditions and less acute major situations. Prevention of disease, health promotion and relief of social problems are other tasks.

Primary care is often the first contact with the health care system and for the patient features are direct access and availability 24 hours a day. The primary physician should become the friend, philosopher and guide of his or her patients, an advocate and protector and coordinator of appropriate specialist services and provide long-term continuing comprehensive care 24 hours a day. The primary physician acts as a health broker.

There is no single prototype of a good primary physician; he or she may be a generalist or a specialoid, may work solo or in a group. Whoever it is, the physician should accept the necessary roles. The work base is most often the physician's office, but the patients' homes and the community must be included. Local hospitals, nursing homes and similar units may be other sites. The work of primary care should be subject to the same scientific principles of critical analysis and audit that apply in other specialties to determine useful effective procedures.

What is Primary Care and Why is it Important?

Ever since human history began there must have been 'primary carers' and healers in the community to whom people would turn for help and succour. It was priests, wise-women, midwives, ladies-of-the-manor and medicine men who provided care in the dark ages and beyond. 'General practitioners' came into English literature in the mid-19th century and 'family physicians' later, before and after World War II, and in 1960s and 1970s 'primary care' appeared as a comprehensive term to include non-physicians as providers for first-contact care. Trends suggest that 'primary care teams' may become the mode in the future (Fry, 1988).

Looking back over the past half century the greatest change has been for primary care to emerge from a cottage industry providing personal and family corner-shop services to big business organizations within national health industries such as the British National Health Service or as piece-workers working with, and for, large for-profit insurance companies in the US.

It is important to understand the general basic features, roles and functions of primary care before going on to compare and contrast the US and UK systems.

As noted in Chapter 2 primary care has to exist in every health system. A succinct definition is that it is the provision of first-contact care by a trained professional, when a person decides such care is necessary, and also continuing care when patient and provider consider it necessary. However, for the future, wider roles and responsibilities have to be considered and accepted. There should be much more to primary care than providing care for individuals when they decide to consult.

Within the community, primary care is in the position to endeavor to improve the health of the population through planned health promotion and disease prevention; seeking out at-risk groups, such as the disabled and disadvantaged, to improve their status; remedy social pathologies; and to collect reliable data on the condition of local communities and decide on priorities. Primary care is the keystone to a health system, a link between free, direct access to the people and collaborating with, and protecting, more specialized services.

With increasing pressure on health care, increasing costs, consumer demand, medical advances and an aging population, primary care's role as a gate-keeper to secondary care is likely to become more important. Currently self-care manages the majority of symptoms. If patient wants and needs increase with a reduction in self-care then there will be further pressures. As many Western countries come to terms with these dilemmas so primary care will take an increasing role. The doctor's role as the patients' advocate may change.

Content of Primary Care

Human beings in similar societies tend to suffer similar problems. 'Common problems commonly occur and rare diseases rarely happen'; this truism is important in understanding the nature and place of primary care.

Taken as a whole, the most prevalent health problems in the community are minor symptoms, respiratory infections, injuries, skin rashes and aches and pains which tend to be self-limiting and self-managed. When symptoms do not

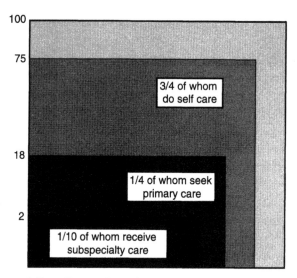

Figure 5.1 Extent of Care: Proportion of Population Receiving Self-Care, Primary Care and Hospital Services in a Year.

resolve or when they are more severe and of possible serious portent then professional advice is sought in primary care. The majority of symptoms are self-managed, only one in four being taken to primary care. Self-care provides for the other three out of four symptoms, with 80% self-medicating. Of those seen in primary care one in ten are referred onto secondary care (Figure 5.1).

Primary care encompasses a true spectrum of morbidity in a community. A generalist physician will encounter all grades of all types of illness and disease reflecting their true rates of prevalence in the population. Since common diseases tend to be 'minor' and rare diseases 'major' the clinical content of primary care inevitably will consist more of minor than major conditions. In our longer living and aging societies there will be increasing amounts of 'chronic disorders'. The proportion of these grades in a developed society – half of morbidity will be with minor, one third chronic and one sixth with major acute and life-threatening diseases (Figure 5.2).

The relative prevalence of these grades of disease is shown in a British general practice in Chapter 6. However, clinical diseases are only a part of the work of primary care as there are personal and family social problems or pathologies to be noted and managed, and health promotion and disease prevention to be encouraged. Socioeconomic factors are important, involving hazardous life styles and the patient's environment.

Most effective improvements in health care occur through application of known preventive measures rather than waiting for 'new cures'.

In a hypothetical district there will be a large District General Hospital (DGH) serving 250,000 people. Primary care is provided by single and group

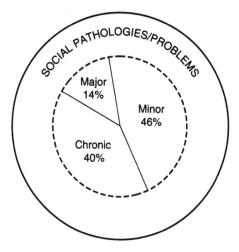

Figure 5.2 Spectrum of Morbidity.

practices and by Health Maintenance Organizations (HMOs) in the US (Figure 5.3).

In such a community there will be primary care provider units. The special features of primary care differ from those of specialist care.

- *Long-term continuing comprehensive and coordinated care* – living and working together in a community, primary physician and patient can act closely over many years and so come to know each other well. In these circumstances primary care is a long-term follow-up process between the same physician and the same patient, rather than the transient situation in a subspecialist practice. Also, it enables the primary care physician to build personal record profiles which provide valuable information (in confidence) to other physicians when appropriate, thus enhancing coordinated care. The continuity of care can be a problem in a system where the patient can have access to a number of different primary care physicians. In the UK the patient is registered with a single family physician. Continuity of care can also be affected in a system where the doctor is part of an insurance plan and is also linked to an employer.

- *Access-availability* – in order to provide good primary care, people must have access 24 hours a day and services must be freely available. Specialist services are best utilized through careful coordination by the patient's primary care doctor.

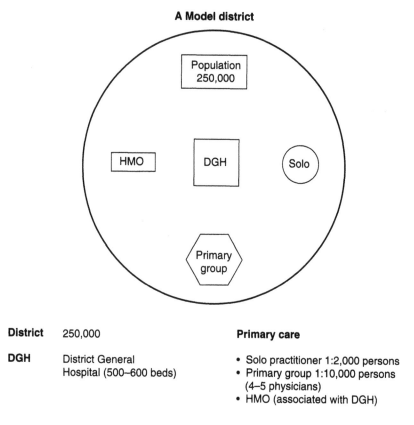

A Model district

District	250,000	**Primary care**
DGH	District General Hospital (500–600 beds)	• Solo practitioner 1:2,000 persons • Primary group 1:10,000 persons (4–5 physicians) • HMO (associated with DGH)

Figure 5.3 A Model District.

- *First-contact care* – this requires particular skills in unraveling the unstructured packages of symptoms that patients bring, rather than neat diagnostic entities. In many primary care situations spontaneous 'cure' often occurs without the symptoms ever receiving a confirmed diagnostic label.

- *Population basis* – in Western societies the population per general primary physician is around 2,000, here the GP will see quite a different prevalence of 'common' and 'rare' diseases from that seen in a community hospital serving a population of 250,000. The population basis of primary care has important consequences for the GP's responsibility for community care.

Roles of the Primary Care Physician

The features of more traditional care are supplemented by certain roles that emerge and become inseparable. With such long-term relationships between doctor and patient, the primary physician becomes a personal friend, philosopher and guide of his patients and their families. The physician has to act as a protector and advocate of his patients from inappropriate specialists and of specialists from inappropriate patients, leading his patients through the medical jungle. This role is likely to increase in the future as more care is undertaken in the community, away from secondary care.

There are resource implications which may limit this development. As a front-line health worker in the community the primary physician has opportunities to coordinate and manipulate available services on behalf of his patients. Increasingly, there has to be attention to the business side of practice, requiring the doctor to have skills of an accountant, manager, director, chairman and politician.

The ambition of a primary physician must be to have the best qualities of a personal doctor while also knowing the patient's family and accepting concerns and responsibilities for the local community. In addition to scientific applications, sick human beings still seek 'tender loving care' from a known and trusted personal and family doctor.

Besides providing a primary care role, primary physicians should be closely involved in providing shared care with specialists for conditions such as diabetes, asthma, some cardiovascular disorders, cancer and others.

From a broad consideration of the content of primary care there are two sets of challenges for the future. The first is to provide personal care for minor, chronic or acute-major clinical problems, for psycho-emotional problems, for health promotion and disease prevention as part of all consultations, and for attention to possible social factors which may be amenable to correction and relief. Second, primary care practices need to accept responsibilities for care of local communities in collaboration with colleagues in clinical and public health fields.

Thus, the essential philosophy of excellence for primary care should be for patients to have access to a family medical advisor whom individuals and families can consult, and who is prepared and able to accept responsibilities and guidance from 'the womb to the tomb'.

Who Carries Out Primary Care?

There can be no monopoly of primary care by any group; it can be practiced by a range of professionals and non-professionals. But whoever does so should note the roles, objectives and qualities described. All health care systems have to include a level of first-contact, primary care, and the strength of the systems depends on the quality of the latter (Starfield, 1992).

The solo (single-handed) primary care practitioner is still dominant in most Western systems (outside the UK), particularly in competitive, fee-for-service systems (Chapter 2). The solo primary physician may be a generalist, specialoid or specialist to whom patients have direct access. Whereas in the past the generalist tended to be a DIY (do-it-all-yourself) doctor carrying out obstetrics and surgery, as well as general medicine, roles now are becoming more restricted, except in remote rural areas.

A move is taking place towards partnerships or groups of generalist family physicians working together with teams of nurses and other professional colleagues (as in multi-specialty groups) (Chapter 6).

A more restricted role occurs when general specialoids provide primary care. A 'specialoid' is trained in a subspecialty, such as internal medicine, pediatrics, or psychiatry, but is then allowed to practice in other areas such as obstetrics and gynecology, but restricts work to his or her population or clinical specialty. In non-referral systems such as the US system, even neurologists, cardiologists, dermatologists etc, have to undertake the roles of primary care, but with difficulties because of their specialty constraints and problems in providing long-term care.

Many non-physicians also provide primary care, such as osteopaths, acupuncturists and traditional healers; here difficulties may occur in managing medical problems outside their experience and abilities.

In many health systems there exist direct access units for persons suffering from mental disorders, sexually transmitted diseases or in need of family planning, as well as many self-help patient groups. Where preventive care is less than complete, access to public health clinics has to be provided for immunization and other services.

The hospital emergency room allows direct access and provides a considerable amount of primary care by default for those persons who have no access to a personal physician. In the US this may be the only access to medical care for those with no health care insurance. Care tends to be on an *ad hoc* basis for immediate problems with little planned follow-up and continuity.

A matter of debate is whether primary (first contact) care is safe in the hands of a 'generalist', or whether modern medicine is so complex that it requires a 'multi-specialty group' even at this stage of triage. However, the nature and content of primary care are such that it is possible for a generalist (as in the UK) to provide safe, effective and cheap medicinal care and preventive and health promotional care. The complexities of modern medicine and specialization often result in a fragmented approach. A primary care physician is able to maintain an overall view of care for an individual and to protect the patient from the excesses of modern medicine. General practice looks well in the UK, despite ongoing internal adjustments, and primary care is in a state of muddled thinking in the US.

The content of primary care is influenced by four factors:

● the prevalence and incidence of clinical and social problems will be that of a practice's patient population; its size and composition may vary considerably

- the clinical content will depend on any pre-selection by the physician. Thus, if he or she restricts work to children (pediatrics), internal medicine or some other field, clearly this will influence what is seen

- the social and health status of the local community will also have an influence on the presenting pathologies, with known differences between upper and lower social groups

- working as first-contact physicians, it is inevitable that many of the conditions seen and managed will never reach beyond the diagnostic category of 'symptoms' because (fortunately) they are minor, benign and self-limiting and a skill of primary care is to accept this and to be prepared to watch-with-care without unnecessary investigations.

It is one of the challenges of primary care skills to untie and unravel the packages of symptoms presented by patients and decide what may be significant and in need of urgent care and what can be observed and reassessed. These and other features of primary care, offer particular opportunities for the physician to develop interests as a researcher, an observer of natural history, a demographer and a social scientist as well as a clinician.

The much smaller numbers of the less prevalent clinical problems however, do raise questions of competence in technical fields such as surgery, obstetrics, pediatrics and medicine. Maintenance of quality and safety by the individual practitioner depends on a sufficiency of numbers of cases to keep up experience and expertise. How many surgical emergencies, difficult obstetric cases and complex medical techniques does a practitioner require to maintain skills? The family physician may only see in a year three or four of each case, eg, acute appendicitis, complicated obstetrics and medical emergencies, compared with the 10 or 20 times those numbers seen by subspecialist colleagues. The answer has to be that the 'occasional' generalist is less experienced. In areas such as these, protocols of care need to be developed by the profession which provide guidelines on the type of cases where a greater clinical competence is required. In the UK the use of maternity units by family physicians is determined by risk-assessment criteria and protocols.

Patients who consult represent the tip of the iceberg in terms of health problems; there are many remediable and relievable clinical and social situations undetected and unmanaged. Future tasks must be to move the front lines of primary care away from the physician's office and hospital into the community to define priority problems and seek planned and coordinated solutions together with other health workers on a locality basis.

Achieving Good Primary Care

How?

The basic principles of good medical practice apply to primary care just as much as to subspecialty care. However, the excellent training that medical students and residents receive from their subspecialist teachers has to be adapted and applied to the special field of primary care. This involves a shift from a disease to an illness focus, with the associated psychological and social components. Other areas include the difference in the prevalence and incidence of conditions, the condition's natural history and the role of self-care as well as non-clinical roles. As a result, medical education needs to be more focused to the needs of family physicians.

With the characteristic features and distributions of clinical disorders in primary care the physician must become skilled more in making priority decisions than in straining and striving to attach pathological diagnostic labels.

These priorities are an assessment as to whether the patient is so seriously ill that urgent hospitalization is indicated and whether the problem can be managed by the doctor or needs referral to a subspecialist. If the patient is being kept in the community, then the doctor needs to assess whether to; do nothing, review, investigate or provide long-term care. In all this, the patient needs to be kept informed and be involved in the decision-making process.

The primary physician's clinical management depends on his or her experience and skills. This will influence whether he or she provides diagnostic investigations in his or her own office; endoscopies, physical therapies or surgery obstetric services.

Whilst personal care on a one-to-one relationship between physician and patient is the crux of all good care the advances in medicine have made isolated, solo practice a feature of the past. For many, but by no means all situations, close collaboration between colleagues has to be readily available. This collaboration has to be on an equal, professional, consultative rather than competitive, basis and it needs to be planned and coordinated. There are many examples where the best care for individual patients and groups of patients is 'shared' between primary generalists and subspecialists with agreed guidelines.

Other ingredients for good care are reliable and meaningful clinical and operational data on which to base future planning, rewards and pay related to priority needs, and audits of quality that achieve accountability.

Where?

Primary care is not an island, but part of a socio-medical complex of many parts, each with their own role to play. Within the levels of care there has to be constant flow of care of patients between professionals in directions depending on needs and circumstances. Figure 2.2, p. 16 illustrates such flows in the US and UK systems.

The flow diagram emphasizes the key roles of primary care not only as a triage filter and gatekeeper but also as an essential front-line operator and as the foundation of all systems.

There are at least five possible functional sites for primary care:

1. physician's office/center

2. patient's home

3. hospital

4. community

5. others.

1. Physician's Office/Center

When primary care was a cottage industry and when transportation was primitive, access had to be within walking distance. In some towns there was one physician's office in almost every block. The office was often part of the physician's home and he was very much part of the local social community, scene and structure. Now, with easier transportation, there are fewer primary care units because physicians tend to work in groups or from special medical buildings. Access for the disabled and young mothers with no cars can be difficult.

In planning a local health system, the siting of primary care units is important for reasons of access and community interaction. In idealistic situations, the primary physicians should be so well known that patients recognize them in the street, and that physicians know these patients by name!

There are arguments for large central sitings (HMOs etc) in order to share expensive facilities and resources; but in primary care this must be balanced against the importance of community availability and recognition that expensive facilities are rarely required and may be more effectively and economically utilized by referral to groups of specialists.

2. Patient's Home

As already mentioned, home visiting by physicians has become less common than half a century ago, when it represented almost one half of their work. Certainly it is time-consuming, with travel and parking difficulties in cities, and few technical procedures can be performed at home, but there are reasons why home visiting should continue and perhaps increase as the number of people coping with chronic problems increases. It offers the privileges of the physician being received into the social privacy of a home; it provides insight into social conditions; it allows the physician to meet members of the family and observe their inter-relationships; it provides social contact to housebound patients; and it demonstrates that a physician really cares and is much appreciated.

3. Hospital

A hospital may be the only access point for persons who do not have the availability of community-based physicians, and therefore hospitals must do more than merely provide emergency facilities. In some communities, it may be that in the future the hospital will become one of the primary care sites and so organize such a service.

Hospital privileges may be available for primary physicians to take care of their own patients (see Chapters 4 and 7), provided they are trained, experienced and competent; that facilities are adequate for unexpected emergencies, particularly in surgery and obstetrics; and that back-up by specialists is readily available. Since clinical outcomes of care in systems with and without hospital privileges are similar, the reasons for continuing such privileges must be the general wishes of patients, physicians and providers. The reasons for hospital privileges for primary physicians include continuity and provision of appropriate personal care at all levels; providing access in remote geographic areas where specialists are scarce; and extra incomes for physicians.

4. Community

As discussed there have to be clearly recognizable, available, accessible and affordable primary care units in the community not only for clinical services but for disease prevention, health promotion and the public health. Should these be part of primary care or set apart and provided by local public health departments? If primary care is to accept social contracts and duties, then it must be prepared to take on these community health roles, including prenatal care, family planning, immunization, child and adult surveillance, and checks and definition of at-risk groups in the community, as well as taking steps to help them. An alternative view is that the present situation should continue with people and physicians free to choose between public and personal services.

5. Others

This includes open access occupational units, health clubs, etc. In the US, worksite primary care centers and school-based clinics are becoming popular.

When?

Disease knows no time scales and services have to be available to provide 24-hour cover, somewhere and somehow. This is quite possible in larger organizations and groupings but can be difficult for solo physicians.

The doctor's day usually revolves around office consulting times and visits to patients in hospitals, perhaps the occasional home visit and other duties such as committees and various outside professional work. 'Out of hours' arrangements for evening, night, weekend and holidays are various:

- the solo practitioner with a small personal practice may try to be available at all times or share duties with a neighboring colleague
- groups can arrange a shift system
- commercial services may be available where unknown employed doctors will see or visit patients
- own arrangements. This usually means a visit to a hospital emergency room and a wait to see any available young duty physician.

Whatever the arrangements some contract has to be understood by patients and physicians and confidence assured.

Why?

A final, but essential, question has to be 'why?'. Whatever we do and however we do it, we should be prepared to pause, reflect, examine, analyse, audit and account for what we do. It is easy to slip into habits and in these days of computerization it should be possible to devise software systems to provide alerts and cautions which apply to ethical, clinical and business methods. In any business there is a need for quality assurance to see if the service meets the requirements of the patients, doctors and management.

Summary

Primary care is an essential level of health care in every health system and is present in both the UK and the US.

The major difference is that in the UK there is a single portal of entry to the NHS through the GP with whom persons register for continuing comprehensive care and who acts as a gatekeeper to the specialist services. In the US there is free choice of physician, and he or she may be a generalist family physician, a general internist or pediatrician, a cardiologist, a rheumatologist, or other sub-specialist. In the US, over half of all physicians are broadly trained, general physicians (like American family physicians), and every resident chooses one to coordinate all medical services.

In the UK, the NHS covers for the whole population, but in the US about one in four of the population has no medical coverage or inadequate insurance. The primary physician has to acquire consummate knowledge of the social factors of his local population and define its state of health and at-risk groups that require offers of extra assistance. He or she has to develop their own personal professional philosophies of caring and responsibilities.

The escalating costs of health care need to be controlled, and only through a strong primary care structure will the inevitable impact of some form of rationing be reduced.

6

Primary Health Care in the UK

Introduction

British general practice has a long tradition. It was incorporated into the NHS in 1948 with its own executive structure (now Family Health Services Authority). GPs are not salaried employees of the NHS; they are independent contractors who undertake to provide primary care for all patients who register with them. Everyone in the UK can register with a GP. Each GP has about 2,000 registered patients. Payment is a mixture of about 60% by capitation, 20% from practice budget for staff, rent and 20% from a range of fees for preventive medicine, health promotion, minor surgery and night visits. In addition, for preventive and promotional services they receive reimbursements of salaries of employed staff and overhead expenses. They also receive pensions on retirement. GPs' incomes are almost at the same level as specialists.

In addition to providing access for first-contact care within the stable communities, comprehensive, continuous and family care is customary. Solo practice has become unusual. Most GPs work in groups (an average of five), and team care with nurses and other colleagues is growing. One quarter of GPs are women, and within the next 20 years the proportion is likely to be one half.

Relations with specialists are good. All specialists work at local district general hospitals and are salaried. There is no competition for patients, but this is likely to change with the development of hospitals as independent provider units. With a closed system of registered patients who have free access to GPs, a strict gatekeeping referral system is possible. There are no 'hospital privileges' for GPs but one in four works part time as a 'clinical assistant' (one or two sessions per week) within specialist hospital units.

General practice is recognized as a specialty requiring a mandatory three-year vocational training period, and GPs are paid for continuing education. There is no shortage of GPs, and their distribution across the country mean that there are now no under-doctored areas. General practice is the most popular field among new medical graduates.

The Development of Primary Care

As noted, primary care has existed since the beginnings of mankind. In the UK the first mentions in literature were in the mid-18th century (Fry, 1988).

General practice, or primary care, was unrecognized as a particular field until 1815 when the Apothecaries Act created the Society of Apothecaries' and distinguished GPs from physicians and surgeons. These two latter specialties had had their royal colleges for two centuries by then and considered primary care practitioners to be inferior. The apothecary-surgeons were generalists who undertook medical, surgical and obstetric care of the people in the community.

The second half of the 19th century saw the development of small community cottage hospitals into which some privileged local general practitioners were allowed to admit patients. By the beginning of the 20th century general practice was established with GPs providing care from their homes and working solo for fees, or for goods-in-kind in rural areas where poultry, fish and other produce served as 'fees'.

As a result of the industrial revolution, there was rapid urban growth with prosperity for a few but poverty for most. 'Going-to-see-the-doctor' was relatively expensive. The first voluntary, self-help, prepaid health insurance schemes began unplanned and simultaneously, usually with well disposed employers' and workers' organizations. GPs were paid either through the capitation fee system or by negotiated, relatively low fees paid by local organizations. The schemes were called 'sick clubs' or 'friendly societies'. The movement spread and was nationalized in 1911 by the National Health Insurance Act. All employed workers below an agreed age were enrolled into a state medical insurance scheme for primary care (but not for hospital care – which was relatively free). Those covered could choose a local GP, register with him, and attend when necessary. Each GP had his 'panel' of registered patients (these GPs were referred to as 'panel doctors'). They received agreed capitation fees and the patients were free to change doctors, and vice versa. Not all GPs came into the system; many in more affluent areas did not, and only attended 'private patients' for fees.

Employees' dependants and families were not covered by state insurance. For them sick clubs continued to provide some prepaid insurance, but most paid small out-of-pocket fees.

Between the two World Wars (1920–1939) there was a growing belief among the public and the medical profession that some type of a national health service was required. One government report, the Dawson Report of 1920, actually produced a blueprint of primary health centers working closely with secondary specialist hospital units, but the medical profession resisted this proposal.

During World War II (1939–1945) all hospitals were taken over by the Ministry of Health under the Emergency Medical Services (EMS) to provide care for the sick and for civilian air raid casualties. Most able men and physicians went into the military but some GPs had to remain in the community to care for families, the elderly and others. The primary care system continued as before.

In 1942 The Beveridge Report was published on public services to be created after the War, this was to include a National Health Service (NHS) freely available to all at the point of service and paid out of a national health insurance scheme funded chiefly from taxes.

The NHS was introduced on 5 July 1948 by a Labor government, with a fiery Welshman, Aneurin Bevan, as Minister of Health. It required three years of bitter strife between Government and the medical profession to reach some agreement. GPs reluctantly entered the NHS, fearful of low earnings. But they soon discovered, in fact, that on average incomes increased and opportunities to provide better services improved.

General Practice – Primary Care

1948–1993

The changes in British general practice over 45 years of the NHS have been profound. From the solo GP working from his own family home, general practice has been transformed into primary health care teams working in groups in the community and providing a range of sophisticated, modern medical and social services. However, the road has not always been smooth.

The 1950s were a period of realization of the poor standards of many general practices, particularly in inner cities. Government and professional committees reported on problems of poor premises and facilities, lack of training and lack of support.

The 1960s were times of turbulence: British doctors were leaving the NHS and emigrating to North America and Australia and New Zealand and GPs were threatening to resign. Fortunately in 1965–1966 the then Labor Minister of Health, Kenneth Robinson, was a conciliator. Together with GP representatives he produced a Charter for General Practice, with much better conditions and remuneration. Group practice was extra-funded, employed staff salaries were reimbursed by 70%, extra payments were introduced to pay for use of GP premises, grants were made available to build and convert, and GPs received allowances for training and continuing medical education.

The 1970s were relatively quiet with implementation of the Charter and increasing popularity of general practice as first choice by students, a major upgrading of GP training by the Royal College of General Practitioners (RCGP), and an increase in pay for the trainees.

The 1980s was a decade of Conservative Government with aims to make the NHS better value for money and planning for major reorganization. The chief factors were:

- continuing upgrading of status and office premises

- upgrading of specialty vocational training

- changes in remuneration and fees to reflect public policies

- broadening of roles and responsibilities through development of primary care teams

- sharing of care for special disease groups with local district general hospital specialty units.

The 1990s are a watershed, strengthening and broadening of GP practices. Larger practices are being given budgetary control over elective specialty and hospital services, community care, home care and prevention. In addition, the basic contract for GPs was revised in 1990 to emphasize consumerism, health promotion, disease prevention, with changes in payment arrangements to achieve these. Larger practices were given funds to purchase and coordinate all community care, home care and hospital services for patients at best prices and quality, with better data collection, checks and audits.

The assessment of quality still is elusive, but systematic attempts are being made to combine 'satisfactions' of consumers and providers with 'cost benefits' and outcomes. Given the common conditions and problems in primary care, this is proving even more difficult than in subspecialties.

1990 Contract for General Practice

In summary, the chief ingredients of the 1990 GPs' Contract were:

- better services and information for patients, including booklets on practice services and staff and directions on appointments, clinics etc

- health promotional activities, targets for pap (cervical) smears and child immunization, health checks and health promotion programs (all to receive fees)

- minor surgery (extra fees)

- deprivation allowances for GPs working in inner cities (extra fees)

- computer grants for practices to set up informed data collection and processing systems

- annual reports from each practice to be submitted to Family Health Services Authorities

- participation in audit exercises

- grants to purchase education (Post Graduate Education Allowance)

- fundholding practices (for internal markets).

General Practice in the NHS

The first principle of the British approach to general practice is that it is recognized in the NHS as a special field of medical work. It has a separate division within the Department of Health. It has its own political representation within the British Medical Association – the General Medical Services Committee (GMSC). It has its own academic representation – the Royal College of General Practitioners (RCGP). All medical schools now have departments of general practice or primary care. Within the statutory standard-setting professional body, the General Medical Council (GMC), general practitioners are well represented and at the local levels GPs elect their own representatives to a Local Medical Committee (LMC) that represents them in dealing with the executive body for primary care and general health services, the local health authority.

GPs have special arrangements with the NHS. They are not its employees and they are not salaried. They are free, independent contractors. That is, they enter into a contract with the NHS to provide general medical services to all registered persons. Everyone is able to register with a GP of their choice.

The local health authority is responsible for paying GPs, for planning and ensuring quality and quantity of resources, for handling complaints from the public and taking steps for hearings for the serious ones and having the power to deduct money from the GP if found to be in breach of service or even removing the GP from the NHS, by removing them from the medical register.

Most GPs work in groups of partners with health teams. There are no billings, but there are many services that have to be recorded and fees claimed from health authorities. Patients do not pay any fees to GPs in fact, it is a criminal offense for a GP to charge any registered NHS patient for a service provided under the NHS.

Costs and Incomes

Nothing is free in modern living, and the NHS in 1993 cost £35 billion ($52 billion), or over £600 ($900) per person. The per capita cost has increased by one third in constant prices since 1975, community care has doubled, and general practice has risen by over 50%, but hospital expenditure by only 25%. Its expenses increase annually, but even so it is cheaper per capita and as per cent of GDP than most developed countries (Chapter 2). Of the 20% spent by general practice, only 8% is for actual general medical care, including physician

Table 6.1 Annual income and expenditure (NHS) per GP (Doctors' and Dentists' Pay Review Body, 1992)

Practice budget	Value (£/$)
GPs' taxable income	40,000/60,000
General reimbursable expenses	20,000/30,000
Special reimbursable expenses	10,000/15,000
Total	**70,000/105,000**
Supporting NHS budget	**Value (£/$)**
Prescribing costs	100,000/150,000
Direct hospital costs	100,000/150,000
Total	**270,000/405,000**

payments, reimbursements, basic practice expenses, fees for special services and others, and 12% is for the cost of GP prescribing. General practice prescribing costs account for 75% of the total national drug bill. The finding of the NHS comes from taxation. In 1991, 83% came from direct taxes and 14% from hypothecated NHS contributions, accounting for 13% of all taxation.

The estimated annual NHS expenditures per GP on prescribing, hospital utilization and income is £270,000 ($405,000). Prescribing costs are over £100,000 ($150,000) and the direct attributable GP costs of hospital investigations (pathology and radiology), referrals to subspecialists and elective non–emergency admissions also are approximately £100,000 ($150,000). Annual income, including reimbursable expenses is £70,000 ($105,000). Up to 90% of a GP's income comes from the NHS based on capitation fees and fees-for-services. The remaining 10% is from non-NHS work such as insurance reports and other duties (Table 6.1).

General Practitioners

In 1993 out of 86,000 physicians in the NHS over 35,000 were GPs. This includes three groups: principals (94%) in contract with the NHS; assistants

Table 6.2 Persons registered per NHS GP

	Year					
	1951	1956	1966	1976	1986	1992
Persons registered per NHS GP	2,498	2,225	2,400	2,301	1,977	1,800

Table 6.3 NHS: Number of GPs per 100,000, 1950–94

	1950	1960	1970	1980	1990	1992	1994
GP principals	19,000	22,680	22,961	26,143	32,850	33,500	33,500
Assistants	2,000	1,335	727	305	250	300	550
Trainees (residents)	450	257	273	1,704	2,000	1,875	2,100
Total	21,450	24,212	23,961	28,152	35,100	35,700	36,150
per 100,000 population	43	46	43	52	62	63	58

(1%) employed by practices; and trainees (residents) (5%) spending their one year in training practices and two years in hospital experience.

The number of NHS GPs and the rates per population has increased since 1950. Whereas the population has been increasing by 0.5% per year over the past 10 years, the increase in GPs has been 1.5% for the NHS as a whole; total medical manpower has been increasing at a similar rate. This means that the list size of registered patients per GP has been shrinking by 1–3% per year, or thirty patients (Table 6.2).

Of those entering general practice as principals between 1980–1990, only half were trainees from vocational training schemes. Twenty-five per cent were hospital doctors who had completed their own approved training programs outside the organized vocational training schemes and 10% were assistants becoming principals.

An important change has been the increase in number of women GPs. In 1950, only 5% of GPs were women, in 1992 it was 27%, and by 2001 it is likely to be 51%. One reason for this is the increasing proportions of women graduating from medical schools and the higher popularity of general practice among women medical graduates.

The number of GPs required is uncertain. A government body, the Medical Practices Committee (MPC) controls the numbers of new physicians being appointed as principals in the NHS and has aimed to achieve equal distribution

Table 6.4 Resident population (UK) distribution by areas of GP list sizes, classified by MPC (OHE, 1992)

By list size	Under-doctored (designated-open) (%)	Balanced (intermediate) (%)	Over-doctored (restricted) (%)
1952	44	49	7
1991	5	76	19

by list size. It has achieved its aims, and there are no under-doctored (GP) areas in the UK. Interestingly, there are 19% of over-doctored or restricted areas and these areas need to be controlled (Table 6.4).

NHS GPs must now retire by the age of 70. Most become principals in their early 30s. So with a professional career of, say, 35 years and with 33,000 GP principals, it means a theoretical annual net replacement number of under 1,000 – but some will die before 70 and others will leave the practice early for other reasons; even if 1,500 need to be replaced with 2,000 new entrants a year there is likely to be a continuing increase in NHS GPs of 500 per year. The MPC has no rigid policies at present and is allowing the extra numbers into the system.

Appointment of New GPs

Because NHS GPs are independent contractors (ie not employees of the NHS and free to run their own practices as they wish) they are able to select new partners. If a practice decides it needs to increase its number of GPs the procedure is: to get approval from local FHSA and the MPC, to advertise in the medical press inviting applicants, interviews and selection by the existing partners. The new partner is then given a private contract with the practice and also with the FHSA and NHS.

Education and Training

All medical students now have some teaching on general practice in their curriculum and a period of a few weeks attached to a general practice. This is organized by the academic departments of general practice in every medical school. Following graduation (five-year course), there is a compulsory one-year pre-registration internship for all young physicians. Specialty (residency) training for general practice trainees is mandatory for a further three years, two years in a hospital and one year with an approved GP teacher. There is a specialty board

(Joint Committee for Postgraduate Training in General Practice) that organizes and supervizes the three-year training period:

- it approves and monitors the two-year hospital component in fields relevant to general practice

- it selects and monitors the 2,500 GP trainers and their practices for accepting and teaching the vocational trainees who spend one year with them. During the three year period the vocational trainees also are supervized locally by appointed GP course organizers and follow a learning program with weekly meetings, research and other projects.

At present there is no required re-certification procedure and no compulsory specialty board certification at completion of training, but most trainees take the examination which has an 80% pass rate.

Continuing education is expected by the NHS and each GP is allowed an allowance of up to £2,150 (1994) ($3,225) a year for postgraduate education to pay for the many courses available. To get the full allowance the GP has to complete thirty hours each year of accredited educational activity in the areas of health promotion, disease management and service management. Currently the system is voluntary, professionally controlled, and there are no sanctions for those not completing the allowance. Over 90% of GPs obtain the full allowance, and most of the activity is carried out in postgraduate centers. This is likely to change as education focuses on not only knowledge but its application, delivered in an active format.

Practices

In the 1960s it was accepted that group practice was better than solo practice, and financial inducements were introduced to promote this. As a result of the Charter of 1965–1966, every group of three or more GPs received an extra income supplement. Naturally this led to larger groups. Whereas in 1952 one in thirty of the NHS GPs worked in groups of five or more, by 1990 the rate was one in three. Likewise, solo GPs are 1 in 10 now, compared to 1 in 2 in 1952 (Table 6.5).

Most GPs (70%) work from their own purpose built or adapted practice premises. The other 30% rent space in 'health centers'. Health Centers were one of the pillars of the new NHS in 1948. The idea was to provide models of units in the community for primary care, disease prevention and health promotion for local people. The premises are provided by local authorities and rented by GPs.

Table 6.5 NHS GPs, % in groups, 1952–94 (OHE, 1992)

Group size	1952	1970	1994(e)
Solo	43	21	11
2 partners	33	25	14
3 partners	15	27	17
4 partners	6	16	18
5 partners	2	7	16
6+ partners	1	4	24
	100	100	100

The Primary Care Team

With the growth of group practices, and following the 1965 incentives of 70% salary reimbursements for staff, there has been the development of primary care teams. Until recently, GP principals were allowed two full-time equivalent employees each. In addition to employed staff, most practices have had NHS employed personnel, from other parts of the NHS, such as district nurses, health visitors and community midwives, assigned to work with patients registered with the practice. A group of five GPs now is likely to work in a team of 36 or more individuals.

In particular, the roles of practice nurses have increased greatly since the GPs' Contract of 1990, when many more health promotional and disease prevention activities were allocated to general practice. Although currently being encouraged, the idea of a primary care team has to be viewed with some concern, and tested, it may interfere with the principles of the personal physician (Table 6.6).

Fundholding

In 1990, larger practices with over 9,000 patients (now down to 7,000), were invited to become fundholders. The fund is to be used to purchase specialist services for consultation, diagnosis, investigations and treatment (including hospitalization when necessary), physiotherapy, occupational therapy, speech therapy and audiology, staff and medication. Excluded are: emergencies, sexually transmitted diseases, maternity and neonatal care, chemotherapy and radiotherapy, renal dialysis, termination of pregnancy and child guidance – all of which are still funded centrally. In 1994 a third of the population was covered by fundholding and it is estimated that by 1995 this will rise to 50%, with 10,500 GPs involved in the scheme.

Table 6.6 Primary care team: estimated numbers and WTE for UK (1991/2) for a practice population of 10,000 and five doctors

	Persons	Full-time equivalents
GP principals	5	5
Employed by GPs		
Practice nurses	3 (part time)	1.5
Manager	1	1
Receptionists	10 (part time)	5
Secretarial staff	2	2
Others	1	0.5
Attached		
Home (district) nurses	2	1
Public health nurses		
(health visitors)	3	1
Community midwife	2	0.2
Social workers, psychiatric		
nurses and others	2	0.1

Funds are negotiated with each practice and averaged £122 ($183) per patient for 1993–1994. These are in addition to NHS capitation fees and any other fees earned by the GP. A fund budget for a practice with 10,000 patients would be £1.22 million ($1.83 million).

If the practice is able to provide purchased services below the negotiated level and achieve savings ('profits') then they can be used to improve services for patients. In 1992–1993 the 'profits' averaged £50,000 per fund (Table 6.7).

It is likely that fundholding will be expanded further, both in the proportion of the population covered and in the range of services. The role of fundholding as a purchaser has had a significant import on secondary care in the market place of health care. However as funding is tightened, there may develop rationing, through priorities, as resources become limited. The GPs role as the patients advocate may be affected as the GP becomes the decision maker on the use of resources. It may be that in the future fundholders combine to have greater purchasing power and include advisors for the prioritization of services. The Government aims to have all GPs as fundholders at one level or another.

Table 6.7 Fundholding, 1991–94

	1991	1994
Number of fundholding practices	305	2,000
(% of all practices)	3	21
Number of GP fundholders	1,759	9,000
(% of all GPs)	75	34
% Population covered by fundholding practices	10	36

GP and Hospital

When the NHS was introduced in 1948, it was decided to separate GP (primary) and hospital specialist (secondary) services. GPs do not have hospital privileges to treat their own patients, and in return all of primary care is theirs. When patients require specialist, or hospital care, the GPs refer them to a specialist doctor and hospital of the GP's and patient's choice. This is usually the local district general hospital.

This was a most fundamental policy decision introduced largely through pressures from the specialists. Since GPs were to be paid mostly through capitation fees, no extra pay was to be allowed for hospital privileges. Furthermore, all hospitals were to be nationalized into the NHS and staffed by salaried specialists (with no fees). It was considered unnecessary and complex to have GPs in the hospital service.

The results were that general practice:

• was defined and recognized as a particular field

• was eventually recognized as a specialty discipline

• maintained the role of managing and coordinating specialty care

• incorporated community prevention and health promotional programs.

Consultants are specialists and subspecialists who have completed their accredited and approved lengthy training of 10 to 15 years (Chapter 5). They are appointed to NHS hospital vacancies by competition through selection committees. Normally, consultants are between 35 and 40 when appointed and retire at 65. Their numbers in each specialty are controlled by the NHS to prevent bottlenecks, that is, almost all in the senior training positions should obtain consultantships. There are few opportunities for successful private specialty practices completely outside the NHS, although many consultants are allowed part-time, privately paid work outside their NHS duties. Their annual basic NHS income is set at about 25% higher than a GP.

There is no direct access by patients to specialists (consultants). Referral is through the GP (gatekeeper) by letter and once hospital care is completed, patients are referred back to their GPs. However, about one in four of GPs work in NHS hospitals as clinical assistants or hospital practitioners for one or two sessions (paid) per week as extra members of staff and as part of continuing education.

Changes in the NHS mean that a great proportion of care will be provided outside hospitals, by GPs and associated community health services as shared care. In shared-care schemes the health professionals are involved in routine management and monitoring activities that have formerly been the province of hospital doctors. Thus, for diabetes, long-term care will be shared between GPs and specialists with agreed protocols, patient registers and regular checks. Similarly, these principles are being applied to prenatal care, asthma, hypertension and other cardiovascular diseases, mental disease and more. Shared care offers the opportunity to alter the balance between primary and secondary care and to question whether secondary care is always needed. Currently it has developed in an uncontrolled manner, and expansion of shared care needs to be properly planned and resourced. The cost effectiveness, patient satisfaction and outcome of different models need to be evaluated. The limiting factor may well be resources.

Referrals to Specialists

There are a number of ways to record referrals from GPs to consultants: one is to take proportions of all visits (attendances) to a GP. Overall only in 5–10% of such contacts does a specialist referral occur. Thus, if a GP with 2,000 patients has 8,000 consultations in a year, this would mean 400–800 referrals. The other way is to note the proportions of the whole UK population who use specialist and other NHS hospital services (Table 6.8).

Since many individuals will be recorded in more than one category it is likely that in a year about one in four (500) of a population of 2,000 will be referred for specialist care. In addition to specialist consultation services, local hospitals provide GPs with full direct access diagnostic facilities. Thus, a GP can refer his or her patients for any pathological or radiological investigations and the reports are sent back rapidly within 24–48 hours. Very special newer technological investigations such as magnetic resonance imaging (MRI) etc are not included and have to pass through appropriate specialist units.

There is another specialist facility – the domiciliary consultation. It is possible for a GP to arrange for a specialist to visit a seriously ill patient at home for an opinion on diagnosis and management. The intention is that the GP and specialist should consult jointly at the bedside. There is no cost to the patient and the specialist is paid an 'item of service' fee by the NHS.

Table 6.8 Annual referral rates for a population of 2,000 (Fry, 1992)

	%	Numbers
Hospitalization	12	240
Subspecialist		
(ambulatory or out-patient)	18	360
Attendance at emergency department		
(usually self-referral)	23	460

A Year in General Practice

To obtain a factual picture of content and activities in a British general practice, a presentation of a year's events is illustrative. As we have seen, an NHS GP has on average 2,000 patients registered. In any one year 70% of patients and 90% of families consulted.

The average face-to-face consultations (attendances/visits) per person per year is three to four. This means that a practice of 2,000, with average patient consultation rate of three, will have 6,000 consultations in a year (ie 115 per week) and that with a consultation rate of four will have 8,000 consultations a year (or 154 per week). The consultation rate differs with age, being 5 for age 0–9, 3 for age 40–49 and 8 for those aged over 80. For the site of the consultation, 78% occur in the surgery, 14% in homes and 8% on the telephone. Since 1975 home visits have reduced from 19% to 14% and telephone consultations have increased from 3% to 8%.

The 1992–1993 workload survey showed that in an average week a GP works 69 hours. This is spent as 43 hours General Medical Services (GMS) (consultations, case-discussion, paperwork, administration, teaching) and 26 hours on non-GMS (insurance work, hospital attachments, committees). Of this non-GMS time, 4–5 hours of it is spent on-call.

Longer hours are associated with; being single-handed, having a list-size over 2,500, being a male doctor, having many attached staff and an elderly population.

Since 1985 the total hours of professional work has reduced by 5%, GMS has increased by 14%, on-call hours has reduced by 29% and each surgery consultation increased by one minute to nine minutes. With on-call services there has been a decreasing trend, with one third of GPs doing no regular night work and a further half make regular use of deputizing services.

In the future, workload patterns are likely to show a further increase, particularly in non-clinical areas.

The volume of work of an NHS GP will consist of:

- 25 office consultations per day

- 3 home visits per day

- 1 night on-call per week

- 1 weekend on-call per month

- 2–3 special clinics each week (eg antenatal, child surveillance).

Demography

Typical age distribution of a practice population of 2,000 is shown in Table 6.9.

In 1991 the proportion of the population aged over 65 was 16% and this is expected to remain at such a level well into the next century. With an aging population and a reduction in those aged under 16, the dependency rate is expected to increase from the current level of 52% to 58% in the year 2025. This will place an increasing burden on the proportion of the population that are working.

A particular advantage of the British NHS general practice is a known, registered, numerical denominator of population at risk by number, by name and address and by age or sex. This allows age groups to be targeted for special preventive care and attention to immunization, pap smears, check-ups etc. A known denominator base facilitates research.

There is a birth rate of 13 per 1000. In an average year there would be 26 births of which 99.7% are delivered in the hospital with 0.3% at home.

- 20 will be a normal delivery and delivered by a midwife

- 3 will be cesarean sections by obstetricians, of which half would be an emergency

- 2 will be assisted deliveries (forceps or vacuum extraction)

- 10 would be inductions.

During the year there will be 5 legal terminations of pregnancy and 5 natural abortions. Of all births 25% are to unmarried mothers, or about six births per

Table 6.9 Typical age distribution of a practice population of 2,000

Age	0–4	5–14	15–29	30–44	45–64	65–74	75+	
%	7	12	22	21	22	9	7	100
per 2,000	140	240	440	420	440	180	140	2000

year. In the UK 1 in 3 of all births is to unmarried partners and has increased from 1 in 10 in 1971. The fertility rate of women now is 1.8 (ie 1.8 babies per couple). The average life expectancy is 75 years, with men 73 and women 78.

Deaths

There will be 23 deaths per year in an average practice population: 16 will occur in hospital, 5 at home and 2 deaths elsewhere.
    The main causes of these deaths will be:

- heart disease 10

- cancer 5

- stroke 3

- respiratory disease 3

- others 2.

Content of the GP's Work

The numbers of persons in a practice population of 2000 likely to consult their GP may be estimated as demonstrated above. However, it must be borne in mind that, in terms of grades of severity of diseases, over 46% are minor, 40% chronic and 14% are major, and social problems may be involved in over one third of consultations (Chapter 5).

Minor

Minor conditions tend to be self-limiting, uncomfortable rather than dangerous, often recurring and for which there are no reliable 'cures'.
    Infections of the respiratory tract, coughs, colds, sore throats, and ear infections are most prevalent, followed by skin rashes, various rheumatic aches and pains, psycho-emotional symptoms, minor accidents, dyspepsias and acute gastro-intestinal infections. Note also the high rate of 'symptoms' referred to many body systems (Table 6.10).

Chronic

Chronic conditions become more prevalent with aging and require long-term, planned care. Their numbers may be smaller but their time requirements much greater.

Table 6.10 Annual number of persons consulting for common minor disorders per 2,000 population

Condition	per 2,000 population
Respiratory tract	
Upper respiratory infections	400
Middle and external ear infections	110
Ear wax	50
Hay fever/allergies	40
Locomotor system	
Backache	120
Soft tissue rheumatism	70
Other aches and pains	40
Gastrointestinal tract	
Dyspepsias	50
Acute sickness/diarrhea	70
Skin disorders	300
Minor psycho–emotional	200
Minor trauma	200
'Symptoms'	300

It is important to note the relatively small numbers of 'hospital type' conditions as Parkinsonism, multiple sclerosis, asthma, diabetes and thyroid disorders because these are considered 'common' by medical students and hospital residents (Table 6.11). Hence the importance to inform and educate that primary care is concerned with personal and continuing care of these rather than episodic care.

Major

Major diseases are life threatening and require urgent measure shared with specialists who have access to highly technological facilities (Table 6.12).

Again the annual numbers emphasize the relatively small numbers expected by a primary physician with a population base of 2,000: 10 acute heart attacks (myocardial infarctions) of whom four will die suddenly, or in a few hours; six acute strokes of whom half will die within a few days or weeks; 12 pneumonias; eight new cancers; six acute abdominal emergencies (of which three will be

Table 6.11 Consulting rates for chronic conditions per 2,000 population

Condition	per 2,000 population
Cardiovascular	
High blood pressure	150
Heart failure (various)	65
Central nervous system	
Migraine	30
Strokes (after effects)	20
Epilepsy	7
Parkinsonism	3
Multiple sclerosis	2
Endocrine	
Diabetes	30
Thyroid disorders	10
Respiratory	
Asthma	50
Rheumatoid disease	10
Other 'arthritis'	50
Chronic psychiatric	55

Table 6.12 Diagnostic rates for major diseases per 2,000 population

Condition	per 2,000 population
Acute myocardial infarctions	
(4 will be sudden deaths)	10
Acute strokes (3 will die within 3 months)	6
Pneumonias	12
Acute abdominal emergencies	6
Severe depression (suicide 1 in 5 years)	10
All cancers (5 year survival rate – 35%)	8
Lung	1–2 per year
Breast	1–2 per year
Gastrointestinal tract	1–2 per year
Cervix	1 in 6 years
Leukemia	1 in 6 years
Brain	1 in 10 years
Thyroid	1 in 25 years

Table 6.13 Diagnostic rates for congenital conditions per practice population of 2,000

Condition	per 2,000 patients
Squint	1 in 2 years
Undescended testes	1 in 5 years
Severe mental retardation	1 in 7 years
Cystic fibrosis	1 in 10 years
Spina bifida	1 in 15 years
Cleft palate	1 in 15 years
Congenital dislocation of hip	1 in 20 years
Phenylketonuria	1 in 200 years

acute appendicitis and about 10 severe depressions with one suicide every five years.

Congenital Conditions

To add to the picture of relative frequency, Table 6.13 shows the likely incidence (of new cases) of some congenital conditions that may be expected by a primary physician with 2,000 patients. Of course these patients will require many years of care and supervision.

Prevention

As well as treating diseases, the GP is involved in preventive care, and in a year will carry out the following procedures for persons in his or her practice of 2,000:

Immunizations	75–100
Pap (cervical) smears	120
Health checks	100
Annual checks of over 75s	120
Family planning	50

The 1990 GP Contract includes specific incentives (financial) for achieving the higher rate of 90% immunization rates of the children in the practice and 80% pap smears for all women (20 and 65), and also for child health surveillance, medical check-ups of all new patients and those aged over 75. In 1993,

Table 6.14 Social conditions of patients in practice (Fry, 1992)

Situation	per 2,000
Poverty	200
Unemployed	120
Divorces	5
One parent families	40
Heavy drinkers (alcohol)	30
Smokers	500
Illicit drug users	10+
Assaulters	5
Sexual offenders	1
In prison	2

95% of GPs received target payments for vaccination, immunization and cervical cytology, with 9 out of 10 receiving the higher rate payment.

Social Pathologies

As a guide to the personal, family and social stresses to which the population is likely to be subjected, Table 6.14 gives numbers of persons likely to be affected.

These social problems are responsible for much suffering and may bring patients for consultations, but although the GP must be aware of them and offer counselling and advice, their resolution is difficult.

Prescribing

It is estimated that over 60% of consultations include a prescription of medication. It is GP prescribing that accounts for over 80% of the cost of medicines in the NHS and 10% of the total NHS budget.

- In the UK in 1992 there was on average 8.7 items prescribed per person (note that over one half of these were 'repeats' when the phone request is met but when no face-to-face consultation is necessary).

- Average cost per item was £7.64 ($11.46).

- Average annual cost of prescription per person was £65.50 ($98.25).

- Average prescribing cost per GP was £123,000 ($184,500).

- Average cost of over-the-counter drugs was £12 ($18) per person (out-of-pocket).

- Top three prescribed groups of drugs were for heart disorders, gastro-intestinal disorders and asthma.

- Generics made up 43% of substances prescribed.

Prescribing is of increasing concern to the NHS managers. This is due to: apparent high rates and costs of GP prescribing that are increasing annually, likely side effects and complications of some medicines and considerable variation in rates and costs between regions, districts and individual GPs. For these reasons, attempts are being made by the Department of Health to reduce the volume and cost of GPs prescribing through providing each GP regularly with print-outs of his or her prescribing content and costs compared with other GPs locally and nationally (PACT). Those whose costs continue to be 25% above average are subject to educational procedures to reduce their costs. Plans are also being made to introduce capped prescribing budgets for each GP and to allow any savings to be used to improve practice facilities. Also the DoH issues 'black lists' of drugs which are not allowed on the NHS and promotes generic rather than branded drugs.

Summary

General practice in the UK has an established role and many advantages. It provides universal access and availability for the population to health care and acts as an effective gatekeeper to secondary care. Changes in health care mean that primary care will be taking an increasingly important role. With increasing management influence GPs will become more accountable for the use of resources and the quality of care provided. This quality assurance needs to be professionally controlled. It is likely that the primary care team will continue to expand and relate more closely to the needs of the local population.

With the insoluble problem of all health needs increasingly being unable to be met, primary care will play an essential role in the prioritization of services.

7

Primary Health Care in the US

Introduction

If 'primary care' only means the care received from the health professional first contacted, then 'primary care' is alive and well in the US, although it is frequently done by subspecialists. But if primary care means care by a broadly trained provider who knows the patient personally over a period of time and who attends to most health needs throughout the life cycle while coordinating other services (ie continuous, comprehensive and coordinated care), then primary care in the US has been underdeveloped for many years. For as Chapter 4 described, within the American system there is no clear role for such a person.

If we add the concept of promoting 'health', the gap between primary health care and the organization of American medicine grows still larger. Only in certain well-run health maintained organizations (HMOs) are services organized this way. Yet primary health care is a key to cost-effective managed care: versatile, efficient, flexible, personal.

Recent History

As Barbara Starfield (1992) notes in her book on primary care, specialization has been widespread in the US since the early 20th century. By the 1930s and 40s many specialty boards had been developed leading to certification for surgeons, internists etc. An American Academy of General Practice was founded in 1947 to promote high standards, although it did not favor the establishment of a board examination for GPs. A board that required completing a new three-year residence and passing an examination was finally crafted in 1969 around the new term 'family practice' – the American Board of Family Practice (ABFP).

This development coincided with the concern about the lack of primary care practitioners that had been raised by three influential and prestigious committees – the Coggeshall, Millis, and Willard Reports. They were concerned, not about first contact care, but about comprehensive, coordinated and continuous care provided by broadly trained physicians. Starting in 1968, many states began to enact laws and programs for establishing departments of family practice or family medicine in their medical schools. (Family practice refers to the practice aspect of family medicine rather than to the academic study, although the two terms are often used interchangeably.) Within four years, 31 departments had been established (out of approximately 110 medical schools), along with 107 approved residency programs.

It is worth noting that family medicine was the first legislated specialty. Medical schools did not establish departments and training programs in family medicine unless encouraged or demanded by state governing bodies. Even now, many private medical schools do not have any organized units of family medicine.

Simultaneously, in the early 1970s, federal appropriations supported a large expansion of medical schools and nearly doubled the number of medical students, in order to fill what was perceived to be an upcoming doctor shortage. The initial grants paid little attention to what specialties all these new students would enter. Most of the new graduates, however, went into subspecialties, so that by 1976 Congress had passed legislation specifically to fund primary care programs.

Many specialties lobbied to be designated as primary care and therefore eligible for the federal largess, including family practice, general internal medicine and general pediatrics. Since 1976, the special federally-funded training grants for primary care residencies averaged only $25 million a year for family medicine and about $10 million a year for pediatrics and internal medicine, compared with almost $5,000 million in Medicare funds for graduate, subspecialty hospital-based training. Although the amount of funding was less than 1% of the budget for the National Institutes of Health, it did provide funds for establishing or expanding much-needed residency programs in these fields.

In family medicine, there are currently (1994) academic units in over 100 of the 130 medical schools and over 400 residencey programs. Although there has been dramatic growth in internal medicine and pediatric residency programs (doubling the number of residents in the past 10 years), most of this growth has occurred in the 'categorical' programs which emphasize preparation for subspecialities. In internal medicine, however, there has been modest but continued growth in primary care (general medicine) residency programs, which now number over 100.

Differences Among Primary Care Specialties

The nature and range of residency training among specialties designated as primary care varies widely, but none so clearly addresses the needs of the community- and office-based primary physician as the training that British GPs receive from the curriculum designed by the Royal College of General Practitioners (RCGP).

Pediatrics is specialized primary care around one part of the lifecycle. In recent years neonatology, or the care of newborns, has become an increasingly important part of pediatrics training. In order to capture the market of children entering the netherland of adolescence and early adulthood, pediatrics made adolescent pediatrics another area of specialization. Most pediatricians train in traditional pediatrics residencies. There are only a few primary care pediatrics training programs. Like all primary care residency programs, they are three years in length. There are also a few combined internal medicine-pediatrics programs of four years in length.

General internal medicine residencies are still much less common than 'categorical' internal medicine programs, and comprise less than 10% of internal medicine residencies. They offer more ambulatory training and emphasize a broader range of experiences, such as dermatology or gynecology. General internists do not see infants, children or pregnant women. About 30% of pediatricians and 70% of internists train in categorical programs and then carry out further training – fellowships in areas such as cardiology and endocrinology. Only 10 to 20% of those trained in primary care pediatrics or medicine programs subspecialize.

Family practice comes closest to training primary health care physicians who can meet the criteria outlined at the beginning of this chapter. Most family practice residencies are in community rather than university hospitals, so that training experiences more closely mirror how they will eventually practice. Medicine and pediatric programs are in academic medical centers, as they depend on university departments for their faculty. This has led to primary care pediatrics and medicine programs producing academicians and very few practitioners. Family practice programs on the other hand, have produced practitioners rather than researchers. Family practice residencies are also three years in length and emphasize office-based (ambulatory) training and behavioral skills compared with the other primary care fields. Family physicians receive training in the care of patients of all ages and both sexes. In addition, primary care does not have much depth of meaning in the American context; it has never been given much credence in the US medical care system and has come to be used as a vague inclusive term to cover the three fields, if not obstetrics – gynecology and the on-going care of people with problems in rheumatology, psychiatry, cardiology, oncology, and the like.

Obstetrics and gynecology training is similar to that of a surgical specialty, and until recently its residents were trained largely with an atypical sample of hospitalized patients. Although they gain extensive experience in doing cesarean sections and hysterectomies, they receive little training in office counseling, dermatology, or musculoskeletal problems. While obstetrics and gynecology physicians are asked to treat a range of problems by women of child-bearing age, their status as a kind of primary care physician is still debated and we will consider them here only in selected passages. Even with a loose definition of

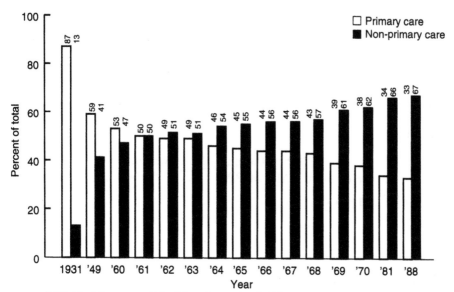

Family physicians, general internists and general pediatricians.
Note: The AMA reclassified MDs in 1968 causing a 3.5% change in primary and non-primary care.

Figure 7.1 A Steady Decrease in Primary Care MDs Compared to Other Specialties, 1931–88. Source: pre-1965 data from Health Manpower Sourcebook: section 14, Medical Specialists, Division of Public Health Methods, USA Public Health Service, DHEW, 1962. 1965–88 data from Physician Characteristics and Distribution, annual editions, AMA.

primary care, only 33% of all physicians are considered to practice primary care in 1990, and only 25% will do so by the year 2000 (Health US, 1990). Figure 7.1 shows the long-term changes in the numbers of the three primary care specialties. There are two important points to be noted. The first is that if one counts all the internists and pediatricians, the US has adequate numbers of primary care physicians and the ratio of 'primary' care physicians to population appears to be increasing. The second point is that the overall numbers are misleading.

Between 1972 and 1990, for example, the ratio of family physicians (FPs) per 100,000 population who provide the comprehensiveness and continuity of British GPs from infancy to old age increased by less than 12% due to the retirement of many old general practitioners, while during this same period, the population ratio of all pediatricians and internists increased by about 75% (Starfield, 1992). This means that most of the growth of American primary care has taken place among specialists who treat only parts of the full spectrum of

Table 7.1 Family physician[1] relationships to managed health care companies by census division, May 1992

	Total (%)
Independent solo, partnership or small FP group which contracts with one or more HMO or PPO	40.1
Member of an IPA which contracts with one or more HMO or PPO	7.2
Employed by a group practice or hospital which owns or contracts with one or more HMO or PPO	14.4
Employed by an HMO	4.4
Other	5.3
No relationship to managed care	26.5
Not reported	2.0

[1]Includes only active member respondents of the American Academy of Family Physicians. Estimates were adjusted by the sampling fraction and the response percentage for each census division.

true primary care, as illustrated in Table 7.1. Most of this was due to dramatic increases in the subspecialty areas.

The proportion of all graduating medical students going into family practice residencies has not increased but actually declined, from 12.7% of students in 1982 to 10.7% in 1992 (AAFP, 1993). During this time, the number of graduating students has increased, reflecting a declining interest in primary care as a career. Although the numbers are harder to interpret because of the mix of categorical, general and primary care programs, there is also declining student interest in general medicine and pediatrics. One basic reason may be the paucity of full-time faculty in family medicine, as graphically illustrated in Figure 7.3. Figure 7.4 illustrates another basic reason: the incomes of FPs have fallen still further behind internists, whose average income has risen because of the inclusion of increasing numbers of procedurally oriented subspecialists (cardiologists, nephrologists etc) in their numbers during the 1980s. Family physicians are acutely aware that the FP's income is only 60% of that of the average physician, and sometimes only one quarter of that of subspecialists, while working the same or a greater number of hours.

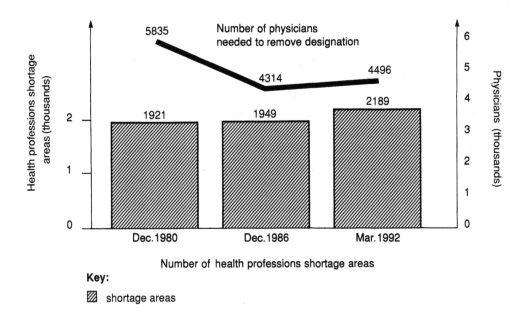

Figure 7.2 Increase in Shortage Areas, Despite 185,000 More Physicians.

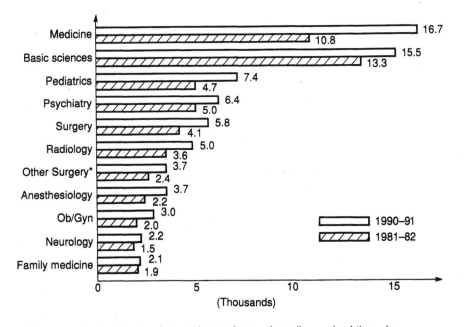

* Other surgery consists of urology, otolaryngology, orthopedics, and ophthamology

Figure 7.3 US Medical School Faculty – Number of Full-time Faculty Staff by Department.

Is There a Shortage of Primary Care Physicians?

As of 1992, there were still 20,200 non-residency trained GPs in the US (most of them older), and 49,600 family physicians (most of them younger). Another 79,800 physicians were internists, probably a third of them dedicated to primary care. The other two-thirds were practicing as subspecialists, primarily in cardiology, pulmonary medicine, endocrinology, gastroenterology, rheumatology, and oncology. Pediatricians numbered 39,700, again with a mix of generalists and subspecialists, and obstetricians-gynecologists numbered 34,600 (AAFP, 1993).

None of these figures reflect a national physician workforce plan; the US has none. As noted previously, nearly all federal funds for graduate training have gone to hospitals for hospital-based residencies ($5 billion through Medicare compared to about $50 billion − 1% − for specific programs in primary care). The number and types of residency positions has little to do with the country's needs and everything to do with the needs of hospitals to cover services with the inexpensive, talented, and energetic labor that residents offer. Indeed, the decision to start or expand a residency is made by the service needs of the hospital, to cover the intensive care unit (ICU), perform procedures, take care of the poor, etc rather than the needs of the surrounding community.

More broadly, no medical workforce policy has guided the number of medical school graduates nor the number of new doctors licensed each year nor the number and type of specialists trained. This has led to an inverse relation between the ratio of problems needing the attention of generalists *vs* specialists (85:15) and the ratio of generalists to specialists practicing (15:85). The large number of subspecialists in the US is a major force in driving up medical costs, a point we shall develop later. Countries with well-designed health care systems have 50 to 60% of their physicians in general practice (Starfield, 1992).

At one per 410 people, the US has many doctors, and at one per 1320, adequate numbers in primary care; but only a third of those provide broad-based primary care comparable to GPs in the UK and comparable to what managed care systems will want in the future.

There are, finally, significant attempts at correcting the imbalance in the US system. These can be summarized as follows.

1. Attempts are being made to correct the inequities in fees through the Medicare's Resource Based Relative Value System (RBRVS) schedule. Other payers are slowly adopting the RBRVS system. The major change that the RBRVS has had is to decrease payments for surgical and technical procedures, often forcing higher out-of-pocket payments for patients. There have been modest increases in payments for evaluation and management services, but because of the historic inadequacies and the fact that the changes need to be cost neutral (with corrections for volume, inflation, etc), these increases have been small.

2. COGME, the Council of Graduate Medical Education, is a commission which has reported yearly to Congress about the need for increasing numbers of primary care physicians. Their published recommendations, to have 50% of all medical school graduates go into primary care fields and to limit the number of residency positions, have achieved wide notice. As of this writing, a number of bills have been introduced in Congress that would make COGME-inspired changes in graduate medical education – including differential medicine payments for primary care residents and establishing national boards with power and authority to limit the numbers and types of residencies. The chances of any one of these bills becoming law is not known; they go against the American laissez faire medical education system.

3. While one waits to see if there will be any federal action, many states and private philanthropic foundations have developed a number of ways to encourage medical students to go into primary care, including loan repayment, increased support of family practice residencies, inducements to practice in rural or urban underserved areas, and model educational programs.

Summary

Although the US seems to have adequate numbers of primary care physicians, if everyone is counted, most of these physicians were not well trained for primary care and do not feel well reimbursed (compared to their UK counterparts). Although not discussed here, there has been a similar lack in workforce planning in primary care mid-level practitioners – nurse practitioners, physician's assistants and nurse midwives. The real action, in the US, has been in the dramatic growth of subspecialists. There have been some attempts, both through reimbursement and through changes in residency numbers, to change this imbalance, but the effect so far is small, if measureable.

Geographic Distribution

The geographical distribution of FPs is depicted in Figure 7.1; in most parts of the US, there are fewer than one FP per 3,000 people.

The number of rural and poor areas designated as health profession shortage areas (HPSAs) has actually increased between 1970 and 1990, despite overall physician supply growing from 157 to 240 per 100,000 population. In 1988, there were 176 counties in which over 700,000 people lived with no primary care physician at all. The lack of access to basic care results in needless premature deaths from such conditions as asthma, pneumonia, hypertension, tuberculosis and infant illnesses.

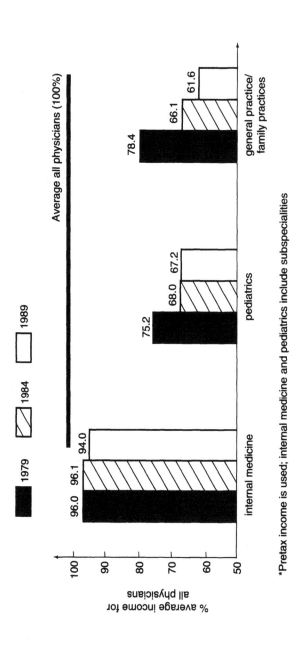

Figure 7.4 Income of US Physicians – Percentage of Average Physician Income for General/Family Practice, Internal Medicine and Pediatrics.

The three graphs making up Figures 7.5–7.7 tell the story of maldistribution in the US. Osteopathic physicians are more evenly distributed across metropolitan areas large and small (Figure 7.7). Specialists, however, are about ten times more likely to practice in large urban areas than in rural areas (Figure 7.6).

Another pattern is that the states with the largest concentration of medical students per thousand population tend to have the worst ratios of family physicians to specialists per thousand population. For example, Massachusetts has one physician per 333 people but only one FP per 6,561. This is a differential of 1:19, one FP for each 19 specialists. New York is not much better, at one doctor per 339 people but only one FP per 5,643, a differential of 1:16, and in the District of Columbia, where Congress makes policy about such matters, there is only one FP for every 19 specialists. At the other end of the spectrum, in Washington State (which has a well-respected medical school with a strong family practice tradition and many family practice residencies), the differential is 1:4 FPs to specialists. In Montana the differential dips to 1:3.7, and in South Dakota it reaches 1:2.4, closer to the ratio of 1:1 which many experts say a health care system should have. Yet no one is championing the use of resources and their quality in South Dakota as a model for the nation. The statistics probably reflect the fact that many family practice residencies are in smaller communities and that family practice residents are better trained to practice in rural areas. Medical schools are located in more populous areas. Nevertheless, rural (and underserved urban) areas continue to experience difficulty in attracting physicians. The great expansion of physician numbers in the 1970s and

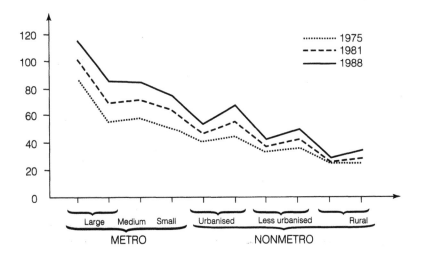

Figure 7.5 Non-federal Primary Care Physicians Per 100,000 Persons by Urban–Rural Continuum Category, 1975.

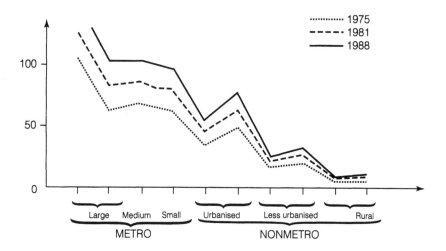

Figure 7.6 Non-federal Specialist Osteopaths Per 100,000 Persons by Urban–Rural Continuum Category, 1975.

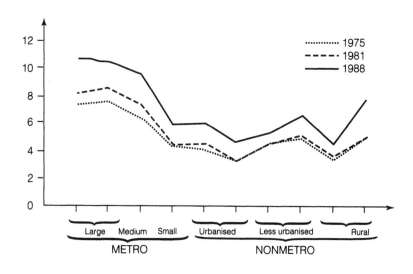

Figure 7.7 Non-federal Active Specialist Physicians Per 100,000 Persons by Urban–Rural Continuum Category, 1975.

1980s did not lead to a corresponding increase in physicians in all areas. The significant income disparities between physicians working in urban and rural areas will have to be addressed in order to even out physician geographic distribution, as the US is not likely to require physicians to practice in certain regions.

The Changing Organization of Primary Care

There is no standard way in which primary care services are organized in the US. Every conceiveable arrangement of physicians is present, from solo practice to groups of hundreds, even a thousand, of physicians; from small community health centers to hospital-affiliated clinics or emergency rooms; from single-specialty groups to large, multi-specialty groups; from those specializing in patients on welfare to those who take only patients who can pay privately; from those seeing patients on only one health plan to those seeing patients covered by multiple plans; and from those paid only by fee for service to those under capitation contracts. These are the products of personal taste, economic arrangements, organizational strategies, and efforts to fill gaps.

Amid this confusion, however, one can discern certain patterns. Starting in the late 1970s, the palpable sense of urgency to hold down the rate at which medical expenditure was increasing produced what has been called 'The Buyers' Revolt' (Light, 1991). Corporations, state programs, and Medicare – as the single largest purchaser of services – transformed themselves from passive payers into active buyers. As described in Chapter 4, they installed hundreds of systems to review what doctors ordered and what they charged. They questioned hospital admissions through precertification review and each additional day in hospital through concurrent review. They raised deductibles and co-payments, and made patients pay cash if they used costly emergency rooms for non-emergencies. They sought providers (hospitals, physicians, laboratories, pharmacies, diagnostic centers, surgi-centers, etc) who would either give discounts for volume or who would accept a fixed amount for all care.

These changes reinforced certain trends that continue to this day. HMOs have assumed center stage as a buyer's utopia: all care for a fixed fee – leave the problems of allocation, coordination and rationing to us. As we said in Chapter 4, they have assumed diverse forms, primarily to broaden their appeal by offering a wider choice of physicians. Hybrid HMOs, PPOs (Preferred Provider Organizations), and traditional office-based practices with managed care features now characterize most practices. In this chapter we will concentrate on the organization and practice economic arrangements of family physicians, as being the most parallel to general practice in the UK.

The Economic Organization of Family Practice

Most FPs either practice solo (this is a decreasing number) or in a small family practice group. Their offices are typically near, but not part of, a hospital.

The most important organizational change in decades has been the rise of managed care systems. The American Academy of Family Physicians reported that in January 1993, only 31.5% of family physicians were receiving only fee-for-service income and 36.5% received their income from a mixture of fees from private patients and contracts with IPA (Independent Practice Association), HMOs, PPOs, and the like (Table 7.2). Contracts now provide 13.5% of FPs' income.

In 1992, the AAFP found that only about a quarter of US family physicians still have no relationship to managed care. The most common arrangements are partial contracts with one or more HMO or PPO while retaining some fee-for-service practice (47%). A small, but growing, number work full-time for a group practice or hospital with such contracts.

With physicians needing patients, who only come to them through contracts, these developments are changing the culture of primary care by forcing doctors to think more like sales managers positioning their line of products to maintain market share. There appears to be an exodus of family physicians with capital and contracting expertise out of solo practice, particularly in rural areas, towards large single- or multi-specialty groups in suburban areas affiliated to hospitals or health plans. Those FPs who remain in solo or small group practices often sign on with managed care systems as a defensive measure, to ensure they do not lose part of their patient panel. Often the first sign of trouble comes when a patient of some years says one day: 'Doctor, I want to stay with you but my employer's insurance will only provide me with full coverage if I go to doctors at Managed Care PPO.'

In addition to the corporatization of primary care, the administrative complexity of plans has greatly increased because of competition between insurance companies. In a zero-sum market, the main way in which plans compete and appear to offer comprehensive coverage at the same or lower rates, is through a variety of techniques that thin out the coverage in previously comprehensive policies. These techniques include exclusion clauses for pre-existing conditions, longer waiting periods during which treatment of such conditions is not covered, internal provisos ('gotcha clauses') that must be fulfilled if claims are to be covered, pre-approval requirements, plus various forms of claims harassment such as losing claims, denying valid claims to delay payment, automatic telephone answering systems that frustrate getting through about claims disputes, and understaffed telephone lines that make patients or doctors' staff wait 10 to 15 minutes before a real human being answers (Light, 1992). Incredibly, there are about 1,200 insurance companies in the US which offer an estimated 50,000 different types of health insurance policy!

Table 7.2 Practice profile of family physicians, January 1, 1993

Practice base:	
Office	89.7
Hospital	7.0
Other (school, industrial, etc.)	3.1
Not reported	0.3
Practice location*:	
Urban	57.3
Rural	26.0
Not reported	16.7
Mean percent of patients whose principal health insurance coverage is:	
Medicare	24.2
Medicaid	10.7
Prepayment-capitation (HMO, IPA)	16.7
Other health insurance	37.1
No health insurance	11.2
Practice arrangement:	
Solo	36.9
Two-person partnership	12.5
Family practice group	32.8
Multi-specialty group 'polyclinic'	17.0
Not reported	0.8
Practice incorporated:	
Yes	51.9
No	46.6
Not reported	1.5
Type of income:	
Fee-for-service	31.5
Contract-for-service	2.2
Both fee and contract	36.5
Straight salary	19.4
Not reported	6.7

*Respondents were asked to indicate city and county of practice. 'Urban' and 'Rural' were determined based upon federal definitions of counties as either metropolitan or non-metropolitan, except in New England and other selected cities where township or city determines a metropolitan area.
(Source: American Academy of Family Physicians facts about family practice.)

These complexities greatly increase the costs of bill collection and require computerization or large fees payable to professional billing services. In addition, utilization and quality review are not coordinated, so that a group practice has to deal with different UR (Utilization Review) requirements and different personnel from several companies, each demanding different kinds of documentation about clinical decisions and procedures. From a physician's point of view, these hassles have significantly increased their office overhead and level of frustration, have interfered with continuity and have complicated medical decision making.

Other Variations in Payments

In addition to the impetus towards managed care, the American system of paying for medical care has other complications. Table 7.3 comes from data collected earlier and from another source than data in Table 7.2 so they are not directly comparable. However, it is important to highlight a number of patterns. First is the large amount (30.4%) of medical bills not covered by insurance plans that patients pay out-of-pocket. Moreover, American insurance policies often cover more of a subspecialist's bill than of a general physician's bill. This uniquely American pattern has historical precedents, such as early Blue Cross and indemnity plans which covered surgery- and hospital-based tests, but did not cover office-based visits. This further mitigates against going to a primary care generalist and motivates patients to guess which specialists they need to see from the start. Overall, this results in more costly, uncoordinated care.

Secondly, payments patterns vary significantly by region and from state to state. To take just one example, in Table 7.3, 13.5% of FPs' income comes from prepaid plans, but this figure varies from 28% in California, Hawaii, Massachusetts and Minnesota, to less than 6% in the rural states like Wyoming, South Dakota, Mississippi, West Virginia, and Alaska (AAFP, 1993).

Thirdly, in interspeciality comparisons, general internists tend to see more elderly patients and a third of their payments come from Medicare. Only one fifth of FPs' income comes from Medicare. The reason for this is historic and demographic. Internists do not see many young patients, so the elderly will make up a greater percentage of their practice and they tend to practice in urban or suburban areas with more elderly populations.

Family physicians see significantly more poor (Medicaid) patients than do the other primary care specialties. Family physicians average 12.3% of their income from seeing Medicaid patients, though this figure varies greatly by region. The reason why FPs are seeing more poor patients probably has to do with their practice location, which tends to be in more rural and urban underserved areas than internists or pediatricians.

Table 7.3 Percentage of office visits[1] by expected source of payment: US, 1990

Expected source of payments	All specialties	FPs	Pediatricians	Internists[2]	Obstetricians/ gynecologists
Total visits	100.0	100.0	100.0	100.0	100.0
Self-pay	30.4	33.9	40.5	29.3	24.1
Medicare	19.8	19.0	0.2	33.0	2.7
Medicaid	8.5	12.3	9.3	7.8	8.3
Blue Cross/Blue Shield	12.1	8.6	8.8	13.9	12.4
Other commercial insurance	24.0	20.1	13.8	23.6	36.0
Pre-paid plan HMO/IPA/PPO	14.5	13.5	26.3	14.0	15.5
No charge	1.8	0.9	0.8	0.7	3.6
Other	5.4	4.4	2.6	5.1	2.3
Unknown	2.0	1.6	2.1	1.6	4.1

[1]Percentages will not add to 100.0 because more than one source of payment may be checked.
[2]Includes only general internal medicine.
(Source: US Department of Health and Human Services, Public Health Service, Centers for Disease Control, National Center for Health Statistics, 1990 data. Unpublished data.)

Practice Patterns

The age and sex of the patients seen by primary care physicians varies significantly across the specialties, as shown in Table 7.3. It is important to note that of all office visits to US physicians, 30% are to family physicians, 12% to pediatricians and 14% to general internists. Visits to family physicians are obviously more evenly distributed across all ages of patients than are visits to pediatricians or internists. Based on Table 7.3, we assume that in the US, more children see pediatricians than FPs: more elderly see FPs than internists (although the elderly make up a greater percentage of internists' practice), and approximately equal numbers of women in the childbearing years see FPs and obstetricians, although above age 45, the majority of women go to FPs. The principal diagnoses of the three primary care specialties (and obstetrician and gynecologists) are shown in Table 7.5.

As in other developed countries, hypertension, diabetes, and common respiratory infections are the most common problems seen by family physicians and internists. This reflects the diseases prevalent in older adults. In family practice, minor trauma and acute illness are also frequent. The high incidence of acute

Table 7.4 Number of office visits (in thousands) by sex and age of patient to selected specialties: US, 1990

	FP	IM*	PD	OB
Male total	81,850	39,085	43,368	310
under 3 years	5,954	319	22,034	67
3–17 years	13,591	2,154	20,512	107
18–24 years	6,007	2,059	315	54
25–44 years	21,593	9,459	256	13
45–64 years	18,545	11,487	202	56
65–74 years	9,764	8,124	49	13
75 years and over	6,396	5,483	0	0
Female total	127,938	57,538	37,780	60,932
under 3 years	6,030	441	17,063	161
3–17 years	15,898	1,629	19,237	1,593
18–24 years	11,770	3,061	692	12,152
25–44 years	38,142	14,079	521	38,414
45–64 years	29,338	16,273	159	6,875
65–74 years	14,466	11,683	70	1331
75 years and over	12,297	10,372	38	406

*Includes only general internal medicine.
(Source: US Department of Health and Human Services, Public Health Service, Centers for Disease Control, National Center for Health Statistics, 1990 data. Unpublished data.)

upper respiratory disease is particularly noted in pediatricians' practice. Because of their older patients, internists see a greater percentage of chronic diseases – particularly hypertension, diabetes, chronic bronchitis and osteoarthritis. It is interesting that, compared with UK rates, psychiatric and skin disorders are less commonly diagnosed. Part of this may be a concern among US physicians that psychiatric diagnoses may lead to denial of payment (if mental health treatment is not covered by the patient's plan) or to stigmatization, since the visit diagnosis must be sent to the insurance company.

Table 7.6 shows the frequency of the types of drugs prescribed by each group of physicians. Antibiotics are the most commonly prescribed agents – in 20% of visits to FPs and in almost 40% of visits to pediatricians. Most of the use of drugs reflects the types of illnesses seen. Somewhat surprising is the relatively low use of psychopharmacologic drugs (antianxiety agents, antidepressants, etc) which comprise slightly more than 5% of all prescriptions given by FPs and internists. Other interesting statistics from Table 7.6 include that fact that hormones or related agents contribute 35% of all prescriptions

Table 7.5 Percentage of office visits to selected specialists by age of patient and 20 most frequent principal diagnoses for visit: US, 1990

Principal diagnosis of patient (all ages)	Visits to family physicians	Visits to general internists	Visits to pediatricians	Visits to obstetricians/ gynecologists
Total number of visits	209,788,000	96,622,000	81,148,000	61,243,000
% of total number of visits				
1 Essential hyper-tension	6.36	10.38	0.04	0.33
2 Acute upper respiratory infections of multiple or unspecified sites	3.93	3.15	7.67	0.40
3 General medical examination	3.33	2.58	5.27	7.56
4 Suppurative and unspecified otitis media	3.12	1.06	12.89	0.11
5 Diabetes mellitus	2.95	6.38	0.07	0.03
6 Acute pharyngitis	2.64	1.48	4.23	0.21
7 Chronic sinusitis	2.62	2.13	2.44	0.12
8 Bronchitis, not specified as acute or chronic	2.60	2.26	2.68	0.14
9 Normal pregnancy	1.95	0.07	0	30.85
10 Sprains, strains of other and unspecified parts	1.68	0.95	0.14	0
11 Other and unspecified disorders of back	1.44	0.67	0.88	0
12 Allergic rhinitis	1.40	1.12	1.80	0.04
13 Health supervision of infant or child	1.31	0.06	15.29	0.09
14 Other disorders of urethra and urinary tract	1.23	1.35	0.45	0.82
15 General symptoms	1.19	1.24	0.46	0.06
16 Obesity and other hyperalimentation	0.96	0.67	0.05	0.42
17 Asthma	0.96	1.23	1.66	0.04

(Source: US Department of Health and Human Services, Public Health Service, Centers for Disease Control, National Center for Health Statistics, 1990 data. Unpublished data.)

Table 7.5 *Continued*

18 Osteoarthrosis and allied disorders	0.94	1.83	0	0.02
19 Contact dermatitis and other eczema	0.92	0.50	1.56	0.15
20 Acute tonsillitis	0.19	0.29	1.46	0.18

given by obstetricians and vitamins constitute another 22%. Cardiovascular drugs are most prescribed by internists, and non-antibiotic respiratory and immunologic (ie anti-allergy) agents are used very commonly by pediatricians.

The lack of a stable, personal relationship between American patients and a chosen primary care doctor is reflected in the proportion of new patients seen in a given year. About 15% of all office visits in family practice and general internal medicine are made by a new patient to the practice, and given that most non-elderly adult patients average about three visits a year to the primary care doctor, new patients make up about a third of all patients seen. This rate is higher than in the UK, and probably reflects patients' changing health plans, changing jobs and moving more frequently in the US. Infants and the elderly average more visits, up to 10 a year. Relations are more stable with pediatricians and gynecologists; it appears that children and childbearing age women tend to stay with them for longer periods. Nevertheless, new patients represent about 12% of total visits to these specialties.

Specific return appointments are surprisingly frequent; 63% of all patient visits to internists end in another appointment, 54% for FPs, 78% for obstetricians/gynecologists, and 47% for pediatricians. Four per cent of visits to FPs and 5.6% of visits to general internists result in a referral to another physician. This probably reflects the broader training of FPs. FPs do no more pelvic examinations, breast palpations, mammograms and other female services than general internists, each of these representing about 4% of all visits.

Office visits are somewhat longer for internists and shorter for pediatricians compared to FPs. The internist's usual visit runs 15 to 30 minutes, the pediatrician's visit length is 6 to 10 minutes, and FP visits usually run about 10 to 20 minutes. In some settings FPs see a younger, and less chronically ill panel of patients than internists which may partially explain the shorter visit length.

Laboratory testing is frequently done in the physician's office; more complicated studies are ordered by the physician from 'outside' labs. Simple X-rays such as chest or extremity films are sometimes done in the primary care doctor's office, but more frequently they are done in a local hospital or radiologist's office. Procedures such as sigmoidoscopy or ECG (electrocardiogram) are usually done in the physician's office. FPs order laboratory and imaging tests about half as often as internists. However, compared to British GPs, American FPs order more ECGs, X-rays and laboratory tests (Epstein *et al.*,

Table 7.6 Number of drugs by therapeutic classification mentioned in office visits to all physicians and selected specialties: US 1990

Therapeutic class[1]	All specialties (numbers in thousands)	Family physicians	Internists[2]	Pediatricians	Obstetricians/ gynecologists
Total mentions (numbers in thousands)	759,406	251,960	149,370	76,370	35,687
		% of total number of mentions			
Antimicrobial agents	125,594	20.06	10.00	39.29	13.29
Cardiovascular-renal drugs	111,125	15.38	26.98	0.43	1.37
Drugs used for relief of pain	77,444	11.89	11.46	3.50	5.14
Respiratory tract drugs	87,491	13.28	9.42	19.32	3.03
Hormones and agents affecting hormonal mechanisms	67,549	7.88	10.53	1.66	35.02
Psychopharmacologic drugs	46,402	5.59	5.18	1.21	1.32
Gastrointestinal agents	31,272	4.79	6.70	1.39	0.82
Dermatologic agents	43,777	4.29	2.23	6.32	8.32
Metabolic and nutritional agents	29,448	3.28	4.27	1.31	22.34
Neurologic drugs	14,140	2.34	1.57	0.25	0.18
Immunologic agents	19,337	1.98	1.13	13.94	0.37
Hematologic agents	9,914	1.03	2.15	0.38	3.85
Ophthalmic drugs	30,704	0.96	0.77	2.08	0.20
Otologic drugs	4,734	0.89	0.71	0.80	0
Other	12,385	1.42	1.13	3.83	0.38
Unclassified or undetermined	43,089	4.93	4.77	4.29	4.35

[1]Based on the classification system used in *National Drug Code Directory*, 1982 edition.
[2]Includes only general internal medicine.
(Source: US Department of Health and Human Services, Public Health Service, Centers for Disease Control, National Center for Health Statistics, 1990 data. Unpublished data.)

1984; Hartley *et al.*, 1987). These differences are attributed to higher patient expectations in the US, clinical training and economic incentives. Table 7.7 describes the tests which FPs do and which they interpret. Tests and procedures are reimbursed well in the US fee system. For example, a flexible sigmoidoscopy takes between 20 and 30 minutes and may be paid at a level of $150–200, while an office visit of the same length is reimbursed at $30–45. As more physicians switch to managed care arrangements, which capitate payments for these tests, the financial incentives will change. The effect of these changes is unclear and variable – for example, blood tests (such as cholesterol) may be done less expensively by an outside rather than an office laboratory. However, doing dermatology or gynecology procedures may be encouraged, as one would lose a portion of the capitation if they are referred out.

If family physicians do many tests or procedures they may also be providing better integrated care with more continuity. Patients may save time and do not need to see as many physicians, and the primary physician is sure to know the result. The key issues in having primary care physicians do a wide variety of tests and procedures are those of training and quality control. Lastly, maintaining skills is often easier if one is doing a procedure regularly and the cost of the equipment can be amortized over a greater number of visits.

Hospital Work

Most US primary care physicians take care of hospitalized patients, which is not true of British GPs. Again, the reasons are due to historic patterns, training differences and contractual agreements. Hospital visits are reimbursed in the FFS system, at higher rates than office visits and more procedures are done on sicker, hospitalized patients. Surprisingly, continuity of care, which is not a cornerstone of the US medical system, may be enhanced by having the primary care physician take care of some of their hospitalized patients.

Most family physicians (84.8%) have hospital privileges and follow their patients into the intensive care unit (ICU), the coronary care unit (CCU), and surgery. On average, while 80% of FPs' work takes place in their offices, 15% takes place in hospitals, and 5% in skilled nursing facilities and home visits. Family physicians do somewhat fewer hospital visits per week than internists or pediatricians. However, the total number of patients they see each week is higher.

Virtually all FPs practice in an office, and Table 7.2 outlines some basic parameters of their practices. However, 85% admit and take care of their patients in the hospital. Table 7.8 details FPs' hospital practice. Almost half carry out some practice in CCUs; 40% carry out some surgery (mostly 'minor' procedures such as circumcisions) and/or are assistant surgeons.

Table 7.7 Percentage of family physicians performing diagnostic procedures in their offices, May 1992

Diagnostic procedure	Perform in office and interpret (%)
ECG	75.1
Dermatologic procedures	55.7
Spirometry	50.8
Audiometry	49.2
Flexible sigmoidoscope	45.1
Tympanometry	34.5
Tonometry	34.4
Endometrial sampling	31.8
Chest X-ray	27.8
Other X-ray	25.5
Holter monitoring	17.7
Colposcopy	16.5
Cardiac stress testing (treadmill)	7.8
Nasopharyngoscopy	7.3
Ultrasound imaging (obstetrics)	4.0
Mammograms	1.8

(Source: American Academy of Family Physicians, Office Practice Characteristics Survey, May 1992.)

A measure of scope of practice for FPs is whether they deliver babies, and most do not. Of residency trained family physicians, only 32% deliver babies in the hospital, and 16% do complicated deliveries (ie those requiring a procedure). Twenty-two per cent do D&Cs, and 73% provide newborn care in hospital except for neonatal intensive care cases (Table 7.8).

A notable pattern in Table 7.8 is that those who have completed a residency in family practice are capable of and do a much broader range of hospital-based services than do older GPs who have had no residency training. The percentage delivering babies varies significantly by region, from 35% in the Rockies to 10% along the East Coast. It is much more common for FPs in rural areas to deliver babies. The regional pattern is similar for the other kinds of hospital work just mentioned, highest in the Rockies and Western Central regions and lowest along the East Coast. This pattern correlates with the ratio of FPs to specialists in the regions. Table 7.8 summarizes these urban–rural practice differences. In urban areas FPs compete against a large number of hospital-based subspecialists. When FPs are given the responsibility, such as in rural areas, they carry out a much wider range of hospital services.

Table 7.8 Types of patient care in hospital practices by family physicians, by family practice training, May 1992

	Family physicians, residency trained (%)	Family physicians, not residency trained (%)
Newborn care	72.9	48.1*
Emergency room (accident and emergency)	72.4	59.3*
ICU (intensive care unit) team	62.3	47.7*
CCU (cardiac care unit) team	56.2	42.2*
Gastrointestinal, flexible sigmoidoscopy	42.5	25.6*
Surgery, minor	41.9	43.5*
Fractures	41.4	34.0*
Psychiatry	40.1	27.3*
Surgery, assisting	38.9	37.2
Interpretation of EKGs	28.8	17.4*
Obstetrics, induction and augmentation	24.7	10.3*
Dilatation and curettage	22.3	20.4

Sample of 1634 residency-trained family physicians and 949 non-residency trained family physicians. Estimates were adjusted by the sampling fraction and the response percentage for each division.
*Statistically significant at $P = 0.025$ using a standard normal 2 test for comparing proportions, a one-tailed test.
(Source: American Academy of Family Physicians, Hospital Practice Characteristics Survey, May 1992.)

Are FPs More Cost-Effective?

Several studies have been done to compare the practice habits of various specialties. Perhaps the best is that of Greenfield et al. (1992), who showed that subspecialists treating the same kinds of patients for the same kinds of problems order more tests and procedures, costing 20 or 40% more than do primary care physicians dedicated to primary care. Within primary care, general internists have a more costly practice style than family physicians (Kravitz et al., 1992; Greenfield et al., 1992; Linn, 1984; Cherkin et al., 1987; Simpson et al., 1987; Strauss et al., 1986; Bertakis and Robbins, 1989; Bertakis and Robbins, 1987; MacDowell and Black, 1992; McClure et al., 1986). The two key differences are (1) FPs tend to have shorter visit lengths and see more patients within a similar work week. FPs may see patients back a little more frequently, so it is not clear if total face-to-face time is different; and (2) internists order more laboratory

Table 7.9 Types of patient care in hospital practices of family physicians[1] by census division and practice locations[2], May 1992

Census division	Total	
	Urban	Rural
Respondents	1,431	801
OB routine delivery %	19.5	36.7*
OB high risk %	3.9	15.0*
OB complicated delivery %	8.0	24.5*
Cesarean sections %	1.2	12.5*
OB UBAC %	10.8	24.7*
OB induction and augmentation %	13.9	33.0*
Dilatation and curettage %	16.7	35.6*
Tubal ligation %	4.5	17.0*
Newborn care %	64.9	64.6
Neonatal ICU %	6.4	8.7*
Surgery assisting %	31.8	56.0*
Surgery minor %	36.0	59.6*
Surgery major %	3.5	11.7*
CCU %	47.1	62.3*
ICU %	53.5	67.6*
ER %	63.5	79.1*
Interpretation of EKGs %	19.6	34.3*
Fractures %	33.0	53.1*
Psychiatry %	29.1	50.0*
GI-flex sig (60 cm) %	33.9	43.5*
GI-full colonoscopy %	0.7	3.4*
GI-full gastroscopy %	0.4	4.6*
Colposcopy %	8.2	12.8*
Nasopharyngoscopy %	4.7	3.8

[1]Includes only active member respondents of the American Academy of Family Physicians. Estimates were adjusted by the sampling fraction and the response percentage for each division.

[2]Respondents were asked to indicate city and county of practice. 'Urban' and 'Rural' were determined based upon federal definitions of counties as either metropolitan or non-metropolitan, except in New England and other selected cities where township or city determines a metropolitan area.

*Statistically significant at $P = 0.025$ using a standardized normal Z test for comparing proportions, a one-tailed test.

(Source: American Academy of Family Physicians, Hospital Practice Characteristics Survey, May 1992.)

and imaging tests per visit than do FPs. Hospitalization rates and prescribing patterns do not seem to have consistent differences. Researchers consistently find that the quality of care, even with seriously ill patients, is similar for FPs and internists (Bowman, 1989; Franks and Dickinson, 1986; Hainer and Lawler, 1988; McGann and Bowman, 1990).

While FPs perform a wide range of the more common hospital-based procedures, they do not use the hospital as often as some subspecialists. Looked at the other way around, physician specialties vary widely on how much hospital business they generate. For example, in 1990 internists on average generated $70,000 in revenues for their hospitals (or costs for payers), and while family physicians generated an average of only $12,000. Obviously, some surgical specialties like neurosurgery or orthopedics generate high hospital revenues, while others, such as ophthalmology, generate lower revenues per physician.

As prepaid managed care comes on line, however, the economic incentives for hospitalized patients will reverse. Minimal use of hospitals will be encouraged as hospitals typically receive a fixed amount (such as $50 per enrollee per month) for a defined number of patients, irrespective of how many admissions these patients have. If physicians are capitated, the current incentives to do more procedures will also change. A hospital in this scenario will obviously do better financially if its medical staff have a lot of family and other primary care physicians who admit patients less frequently. This situation is particularly crucial in the new Medicare HMOs where the number of hospital days per 1,000 enrollees per year is now around 2,500, and must be lowered to 1,500 or less for the managed care plan to be economically successful. Under prepaid care, an integrated hospital or medical care system must consider the primary care multiplier effects. Each dollar billed by the primary care physician will generate another $5 or $6 expenses to the overall system for pharmacy, laboratories, subspecialty consultations and hospitalizations. Therefore, if a hospital-affiliated clinic adds a family physician, who then sees 1,500 new capitated patients, the physician may generate $200,000–300,000 in expenses or capitated payments. All the providers in that physician's referral system will generate well over $1.5 million a year in new charges or payments. Thus, in the current market, each hospital or large group is forming alliances with other providers and recruiting primary care physicians in order to increase its primary care capacity.

US-UK Comparisons Between FPs and GPs

It is interesting to conclude with some comparisons between primary care in the US and the UK. Table 7.10 gives the numbers of direct patient visits (consultations) in a typical week for a US family physician and a British GP. British GPs see 20% more patients and make ten times more home visits but make only one-tenth as many visits to their hospitalized patients. This reflects the

Table 7.10 Estimated numbers of consultations per week for US family physician and UK general practitioner

	US (AAFP, 1991)	UK (Fry, 1992)
Office consultations	108	131
Home visits	2	20
Hospital patients and visits to nursing homes	26	3
Totals	136	154

much stricter organizational division in the UK between hospital-based and office-based medicine. As in many countries, office-based physicians do not have hospital privileges. On the other hand, they have a clear role in the health care system and do not face competition from hospital-based specialists. This trade-off between hospital continuity versus home care continuity is based primarily on economic issues; however, it reinforces US family physicians' orientation towards sick patients and procedures while British GPs become more oriented towards prevention and health maintenance.

US family physicians work long hours and many more hours a week than their British counterparts (56 *vs* 42) (Table 7.11). The British think they are faster and more efficient, treating more patients in less time with no difference in quality. Americans tend to think that short British visits mean lower quality, but there is little systematic evidence to support this. Ironically, in the UK, the average list size (the number of people a GP is responsible for) is creeping downward from approximately 2,200 to 1,800, which indirectly acknowledges that GPs need to spend more time with patients. In US managed care systems, FPs are also responsible for about 2,000 patients.

Both US and UK doctors write a prescription during two-thirds of their patient visits for one or more drugs. But American doctors prescribe nearly twice as many drugs per patient at nearly twice the cost. Ironically, British policymakers feel more intensely than their American counterparts that pharmaceutical costs are spiraling out of control (Table 7.12).

Table 7.12 provides more detail, not only on prescribing but also on procedures, referrals and hospitalizations. American physicians carry out far more procedures, but refer fewer patients to subspecialists than do UK GPs. This probably reflects the organization of budgets and incentives in the two countries. GPs are on a capitated basis, but consultations and hospitalizations are charged to the District Health Authority's budget. Therefore, until the recent reforms, there was no incentive for the GP not to refer a patient. As both

Table 7.11 Weekly hours worked by US family physician and UK general practitioner

Hours per week	US (AAFP, 1991)	UK (Fry, 1992)
Direct patient care	48	37
Other professional duties	8	5
Total	56	42

Table 7.12 Annual per person expenditure on pharmaceuticals (OHE, 1992)

Country	Annual pharmaceutical expenditure per person (prescribed and non-prescribed) (1990)		Annual number of prescription items per person (1989)
	£	($)	(estimate)
Japan	198	(300)	50
France	112	(168)	36
USA	110	(165)	17
Switzerland	106	(160)	8
West Germany	91	(136)	13
Sweden	77	(115)	6
UK	64	(96)	8
Denmark	61	(92)	7
The Netherlands	53	(80)	4

systems move towards prepaid contracts under a single budget for all services, the differences in Table 7.12 will probably diminish (Light and May, 1994).

The practice of obstetrics, though not strictly primary care, illustrates another difference in costs and style between the two systems. As Table 7.13 shows, the British have far more nurse-midwives and far fewer obstetricians and gynecologists. The specialists deal largely with the relatively small proportion of cases too complicated for the nurse-midwives. Britain is one of several countries that use nurse-midwives extensively, and as the US becomes serious about its extraordinary medical costs, it may follow this example. In the US FPs, particularly in rural areas, deal with most of the uncomplicated deliveries and most family practice residency programs see this as a crucial aspect of their training. To date in the US, nurse-midwifery practice has not been supported directly or indirectly by the medical profession, and there are few funds to support their training programs. More broadly, GPs in Britain have much more institutional,

Table 7.13 Comparison of work in US and UK primary care (AAFP, 1991; Fry, 1992)

Prescribing	US	UK
% consultations with prescription	70	60
Cost of prescriptions per person per year	$154 (£103)	$99 (£66)
Procedures (% consultations)		
BP check	47	15
Urine test	13	10
Blood test	40	10
ECG and other	22	5
Referral to subspecialist	2.5–5	5–10
% Population hospitalized per year	14	12

cultural and financial support than do FPs in the US. They have a clear and uncontested role in the health care system; they work closely with nurse-midwives and obstetricians, not in competition with them. The social and professional status of GPs is quite high, and it is the first choice of many young graduates. More than half of the 3,750 medical school graduates each year sign up for the general practice training programs.

Income differentials with specialists are much less in the UK than in the US. Total lifetime career earnings of GPs are only 15–20% lower than those of subspecialists, compared to being 50–80% lower in the US. Moreover, British GPs start earning full incomes several years earlier than do those still training for subspecialties. This may be an important factor in some physicians' choice of career – having a high income earlier when one is starting one's own family. However, once in practice, some subspecialties are able to do part-time private practice and are more likely to receive large bonuses from merit awards, so that some subspecialists earn considerably more than GPs.

Although US primary care physicians appear to earn considerably more than British GPs, the latter have many benefits. While US FPs averaged about $100,000 in personal gross income in 1992, GPs made about $75,000. However, the GP also gets an additional 14% towards a pension fund which pays a retirement income indexed to inflation. This means that during 20–30 years of retirement, inflation never eats away the value of an NHS pension. Moreover, GPs get considerably more perks besides the excellent retirement system, including free medical education (there is no medical student debt), extra funds for continuing education, and low malpractice costs. Although their take home pay may be more, US physicians must often pay off all training debts, pay for malpractice insurance, and hope that their retirement income does not dwindle too quickly. Since British GPs are assured of their annual contract for their practice (competition being minimal by American standards) and their inflation-

Table 7.14 Obstetricians and nurse-midwives, US and UK – numbers and rates per population

	US (Board certified)	UK (Consultants and board certified registrars)
Obstetricians		
Numbers	31,000	1,350
1 per population	1 per 8,070	1 per 42,560
Nurse-midwives		
Numbers	4,000	24,500
1 per population	1 per 62,500	1 per 2,347

proof retirement income, they are quite well off. And, of course, all medical care for them and their families, as British residents, is free for life at the point of delivery!

Summary

The patterns of primary care in the US describe a piecemeal, uncoordinated system left to the 'free' enterprise of physicians and patients. However, there is a rapid transition of medical insurance plans in many parts of the country. HMOs bring an increased emphasis on 'primary' care, but this has been more a change in finance than organizational culture. Clinical care for patients in these plans is good, but tends to be done by physicians in relative isolation.

American primary care physicians are forced to respond more to the expectations of patients and the terms of medical insurance plans than to the standards of colleagues; the American emphasis on complete patient choice means that lay people make many of the decisions about whom they should see about what.

Combined with high patient expectations for technological cures and strong financial rewards for using this technology, Americans and their physicians have de-emphasized primary care, only to find that it is now the key to making a medical care system work effectively and efficiently.

Compared to the UK and some other nations, the American clinical system makes little attempt to feel responsible for local communities in prevention, health promotion, or community care. Community wide collaboration of services across specialties for the needs of people with chronic disorders, drug and alcohol problems, or psychiatric disorders is rarely done except on an *ad hoc* basis.

All this will change as medical plans budget on a risk-adjusted capitated basis as part of national health care reform. It is crucial that American providers and policymakers study and appreciate the British primary care model in order to understand the changes that need to be made.

8

Primary Managed Care: 'More Choice and Less Cost'

Fundamental reforms of the American health care system are underway to attain both universal access and high quality care at reasonable cost. Britain's National Health Service, Germany's famed system of private and public services, Sweden's socialist system, New Zealand's health care system, and others have attained all three of these goals for years and yet are also in the throes of basic reform. In this chapter we will concentrate on the US reforms now underway.

Some thoughtful observers say that it is impossible to attain all three goals and that expenses can only be held down through rationing (Schwartz, 1987; Aaron and Schwartz, 1993; Light, 1992b). Ultimately, they are right. But a great deal of overcharging and inefficiency should be eliminated first before we start denying services to anyone. Very good health care systems like Germany's or Sweden's or France's (each quite different from the other) have for years been managing all the medical problems of all citizens promptly for 8 to 9% of GNP by avoiding the high charges and profits that make every aspect of American medicine so costly. The US can come close to doing the same.

For the sake of the nation's economy and competing social services like education, the target of US health reform should be to reduce health expenditures to 10% of GNP. This may seem wholly unrealistic, but in this concluding chapter we frame out just such a budget. Ten per cent of GNP is possible by cutting down on the overuse of expensive technology, eliminating inefficiencies in the too complicated organization of care, and reducing the high mark-ups and profits that make the American health care so much more expensive than similar care in other affluent nations. But the heart of the solution lies in developing a strong, expanded primary care model of services that integrates nursing, community care and public health with general medicine.

Illusions of Quality in the Current System

Many policy leaders emphasize that the American health care system is 'the best in the world', a boast not accepted by any policy leader we know outside the

US. The claim is usually substantiated by referring to the world-class centers where superspecialty procedures are done on the most subtle and difficult technical problems. These are indeed among the best in the world, but they are a narrow form of quality involving one patient in 10,000.

A group of concerned clinicians has developed what we think is a much broader and more thoughtful framework for defining quality of health care (Physicians for a National Health Program, 1993). It begins with access. Without universal access and equal access regardless of income, ethnicity, age, employment or insurance status, quality is deeply compromised. The golden rule of health care is that if a service is necessary or beneficial for oneself, it is so for others too (Eddy, 1991).

Continuity of care around a personal primary care doctor, shared medical records, and a team approach to continuous quality improvement, form another cluster of criteria for quality that are largely lacking in the present medical system. Their absence underlies many of the complaints and mishaps among middle-class and affluent Americans. Table 8.1 lists the basic problems of quality that are much more pervasive in US health care than are world-class centers of superspecialty medicine. Each has been fully documented in professional reports and evaluation research. Together, they produce far more medical problems, expense and unhappiness than 'best in the world' medicine solves and none of them can be solved by 'best in the world' strategies.

The quality of American health care can be significantly improved through a combination of national and regional budgeting that provides the appropriate number and kinds of providers and facilities, together with a financially neutral team approach to treating both community and patient needs. This differs from the CQI (continuous quality improvement) programs so popular now with large managed systems in two basic ways. CQI programs divert attention from the systemic sources to poor quality and inequality by defining quality only in terms of operational detail. And CQI programs are often used by management in ways that increase stress, make the playing field less level, make rewards more unequal to control health providers, and reduce clinical work to measurements, rather than being used in an egalitarian and flexible way (Schiff and Goldfield, 1994). The deeper goals of CQI programs may include increasing profits, eliminating jobs, and disempowering workers.

From Specialized Medical Care to Primary Health Care

A high-quality health care system may reduce inefficiencies and high charges through a managed competition, but what pushes costs up so steeply is the paradigm of specialized, high-tech medicine that treats the illness of single organs with the most advanced techniques and thorough regimens possible. Prevention, public health, primary care and community health programs are at

Table 8.1 Problems of quality in the American health care system

- Denial of care and discrimination
- Fragmentation, discontinuity, lack of shared records
- Maldistributions by area and specialty
- Unnecessary tests, procedures and surgery
- Inappropriate and overprescribing
- Iatrogenesis (diseases, accidents caused by medical care)
- Distrust, declining satisfaction
- Lack of preventive and prenatal care
- Lack of comprehensive, coordinated, continuous primary care
- Inappropriately trained, incompetent, or impaired providers

the outer edge of this paradigm. Yet 60% of all illness and death today may be prevented or postponed (PEW Health Professions Commission, 1991). Thus, we are spending most of our money at the far end of the health–disease–death continuum.

The paradigm shift we urge is the same one perceived by Edward O'Neil, the executive director of the PEW Commission, as he has been analyzing trends in American medicine (Physicians for a National Health Program, 1993). Eight trends that characterize the shifts in American health care are as follows:

From a focus on	*To a focus on*
Specialized care	Primary care
Hospital care	Ambulatory/community care
Acute care/cure	Prevention/illness management
Individual patients	Populations/communities
Individual providers	Provider teams
Professionally governed	Managerially governed
No budget/weak controls	Global budget/strong controls
Voluntary coverage	Universal coverage

We should have no illusions, however, about how deeply we are immersed in the old paradigm. Employers pay the equivalent of half of all corporate pre-tax profits for health insurance premiums. Nationally, expenditures for medical services consume 50% more of the nation's gross income than other affluent nations with excellent services, and twice as much as the UK spends with its rationing of elective procedures.

This alternate paradigm to medical and surgical intervention once pathology is manifest, starts at the other end. It aims to maximize health and functioning by moving upstream to the sources of disease, disability and death. First, one must guarantee everybody such rudiments as uncontaminated fresh food, clean weatherproof housing, safe water, clean air, safe neighborhoods, and safe working conditions. Even in America in the 1990s, these rudiments are not securely in place for millions of citizens, and numerous studies show that people weakened or made vulnerable by lacking these rudiments get sicker or die earlier as a result (Aday, 1993). As President Clinton emphasized in his opening address on national health care reform, preventable illness that takes a high personal and financial toll on people can be avoided (Clinton, 1993).

In order to maximize health and functioning, both primary and secondary prevention must receive greater financial support and clinical emphasis. Primary prevention means preventing health problems before they develop, and includes immunizations, well-child care, occupational safety programs, drug and alcohol prevention programs, anti-violence campaigns, and good family planning. Secondary prevention means diagnosing diseases at their asymptomatic stage and before the development of symptomatic illness or disability.

Integral to effective primary and secondary prevention is community-based primary care, the foundation for any cost-effective delivery system. This may seem obvious but it is largely ignored in the US as both reformers and providers focus on developing large delivery systems to prepare for 'managed competition'. Their preparations, ironically, may minimize the successful implementation of a cost-effective delivery system.

Primary care, as we have indicated, includes the treatment of most acute and chronic health problems, in the office, in the home or nursing home, in the hospital, and in critical care settings (AAFP, 1993). It includes triage, counseling, patient education, health maintenance, and health promotion as well as disease prevention. It is best provided by physicians trained in these skills for anyone with an undiagnosed sign, symptom or health concern.

Let us make clear that the 'managed' in managed care is different to the 'managed' in managed competition. The latter refers to an independent person or body managing the market in order to make competitors (ie large insurance companies' managed health plans) focus on efficiency, effectiveness and value for money, rather than on avoiding the sick or undertreating them as a way to compete. By contrast, managed care refers at its core to clinicians orchestrating the various tests, treatments, and services for a patient with a complicated problem. Case managers are non-physicians, usually employed by a hospital or HMO, who work with a patient, the family and the physician to find more effective and less costly ways to meet the multiple needs of patients with complicated problems.

When the term 'managed care' refers to setting up corporate conglomerate of services, the term is already losing sight of its clinical essence. One hopes that a good management team has the patients' best care uppermost in their minds. However, they may equally have in mind balancing clinical management against their debt service or return to their investors. This is the great danger in using the term 'managed care' at the organizational or corporate level. 'Managed care system', therefore, comes close to being Orwellian newspeak that tries to make people think that a multi-million dollar business complex is simply an extension of one's personal physician.

Let us clarify also that by 'community-based primary care' we do not mean any doctor in a community who does first-contact medicine. A housewife with an arthritic hand who goes directly to a nearby rheumatologist is not an example of community-based primary care, and her act does not make the rheumatologist a primary care doctor. We mean much more, as set out in Chapter 1. A primary care doctor is a person who is broadly trained to diagnose and treat 80 to 90% of the problems that people of all ages bring to the office, and who is the patient's personal physician over time. Skills in managing common diseases, patient education and prevention, continuity of care, and clinical coordination are the real money-savers.

Continuity of Care is Crucial

Continuity of care is the cornerstone of primary care and cost management. In a study of low-income pregnant women on Medicaid, for example, those who did not receive prenatal coordinated care services were 21% more likely to give birth to low birthweight babies and 62% more likely to have very low birth-weight babies (Buescher et al., 1991). The infant mortality rate was 23% higher than among women receiving prenatal coordinated care services. Patients who are old, black or poor are the most likely to lack continuity of care (Moy and Hogan, 1993; St Peter et al., 1992).

Studies document the value physicians place in knowing patients well, and their accumulated knowledge plays an important part in their decision making and sense of responsibility to patients (Hjortdahl, 1991, 1992). It almost seems too obvious to mention that when doctors know their patients over a period of time, they are more able to anticipate what problems might arise. They are more able to intervene earlier in the disease process, they have more influence with patients in persuading them to take certain measures, they need fewer tests, they can coordinate specialty services more effectively, and they can do more with home care, self-care and family care because they know the patient's situation better. If all this is obvious, it is equally obvious that competition intentionally breaks down continuity of care. Continuous, coordinated primary care is incompatible with competition.

Patients value continuity of care. In a recent study, when a Medicare HMO dropped a medical group, 60% of its patients left the HMO and followed the group to another delivery system (Sofaer and Hurwich, 1993). Personal, continuous care significantly affects patient satisfaction (Hjortdahl and Laerum, 1992; Blankfield *et al.*, 1990; Gabel *et al.*, 1993). The very kind of impersonal primary care that many HMOs and multispecialty groups are developing to replace personal, primary care doctoring, receives significantly lower ratings from patients (Rubin *et al.*, 1993). Yet corporate and commercial forces are forcing millions of people to lose the former for the latter.

Why Managed Competition Will Not Work

The current proposals for managed competition do go quite some way towards realigning incentives to focus on prevention and illness management of defined populations within a fixed budget. The main problem, however, is that the care will be discontinuous and managed by huge corporate systems. Already the major hospital and medical systems in many parts of the country are buying, merging, and building large, vertically integrated systems so that they will be the dominant managed care system in their area.

This bodes ill for doctors and patients, both of whom approach health care as a small, local, personal service. It maximizes administrative and marketing costs, especially if the extra layer of insurance companies make a profit by being the middlemen or the managed-system broker. Competition breaks up the only proven way to maximize health and quality while minimizing costs – coordinated, continuous, comprehensive primary care. This is the elementary point that businessmen and conservatives need to face in their enthusiasm for competitive health care.

Reform proposals that encourage people to shop for the best plan and be bombarded with inducements to switch each year undermines the very features of good primary care that save the most money. Under several of the current reform proposals, doctors will belong to various, corporately managed systems, each vying for next year's business. Competing plans vye for the patients who least need medical services. Each has their own proprietary clinical records and computer systems. Each year an employer may change the plans offered, or a given plan may change the doctors with whom it contracts, or patients may change plans. Thus change, not continuity, occurs at every level. If patients change primary care doctors, the doctors will not be able to share information about the patients easily. They will not know the patient well, and it will not be in their interest to do so if the patient is likely to change doctors or plans again, or if the plan is likely to drop these doctors for others.

Moreover, management in the front office will encourage giving as few services as possible, or at least as inexpensive care as possible during the contract year, because in the following year the patient may switch plans, or the managed care system may lose its contract covering the patient. Instead of a community of clinicians looking after a community of people, managed competition creates a climate of fragmentation and short-sighted behavior focused on this year's contract.

The evidence suggests that HMOs reduce hospital utilization, and if they do save money, it is primarily from reduced admissions to in-patient care. Whether competing HMOs further lower hospital use is debatable (Aaron and Schwartz, 1993; Fielding and Rice, 1993; Rice et al., 1993).

The proposed structure of managed competition will ironically minimize competition, first because if physicians are in several plans they will essentially compete against themselves, and second because in most markets there are not enough people to support a number of competing managed care plans.

Figure 8.1 shows the areas of the US that researchers have concluded would support three or more plans. Clearly, in most of the nation the proposed structure will lead to monopolies. Even five systems constitutes an oligopoly, where price competition is minimal and the plans divide up the market between them. Thus true competition is possible between large managed systems in even fewer areas than in Figure 8.1. Managed competition also adds substantial costs for extra management, marketing and monitoring.

Much larger cost-savings lie further upstream in the office of a doctor who knows the patient well, can diagnose with fewer tests, is much less likely to 'find' pathology in the first place, and if it is there, knows the patient has responded to previous interventions. Comprehensive, continuous, coordinated and accessible care leads to more early diagnoses and more appropriate responses at lower costs. Without that, US reform aimed at managed competition is slated to institutionalize fragmented care, costly care. Our generalist version of primary care needs to be community based; so many risk factors operate at this level and many people's health problems can be attended locally. This is especially true of those with functional limitations and chronic disorders; treating them in a specialized medical setting costs much more and is less effective. Large institutional approaches for the elderly for those with mental illness, or those with AIDS are extremely expensive and may be needed only for those with the most profound problems. Community outreach and taking care of people in their usual surroundings is a much more common feature of British primary care.

To summarize, managed competition between a few large vertically integrated delivery systems, especially if run in order to maximize financial profits for their investors, is seriously flawed in its design. It depends on shopping and switching, which breaks up the continuity of care that is so vital for lower costs and higher quality. It discourages coordination of care, except among the providers and institutions that belong to a given system in a given year. It commercializes health services, treating them explicitly as a commodity in hopes that the invisible hand of self-interest will benefit society as a whole. And yet the competition has to be heavily managed precisely because competition in medicine is

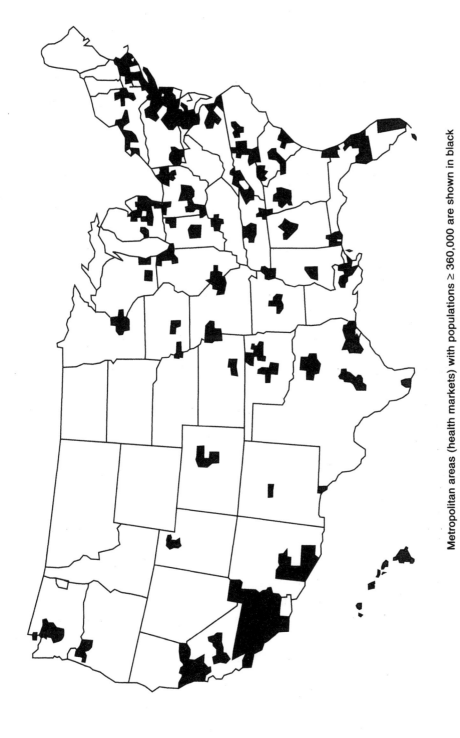

Metropolitan areas (health markets) with populations ≥ 360,000 are shown in black

Figure 8.1 Areas With Sufficient Population Density to Support Three or More Managed Care Systems in the US.

known to harm society in so many ways (Enthoven, 1988). Five of the most experienced and distinguished health economists reviewed proposals for competing health insurance plans and concluded from the evidence that competition, despite its theoretical attractions in some types of economic activity, can easily offend against both efficiency and equity principles in the case of insurance. In Germany, even the competition between the Sickness Funds has led to adverse selection, with increasing numbers uninsured, and rising administrative costs (Cuyler, 1991).

Competing delivery systems require large overhead costs with highly paid executive staff, and medical markets require large transaction costs. Such systems are not particularly interested in the health needs of vulnerable populations or the public as a whole. Finally, they discourage or even break up community-based networks and programs to improve health and make people more self-sufficient.

Primary Care as the Key to Managed Care

The bedrock of good managed care (whether in a large regional or small local system) is good primary care. The following are six key concepts for a well-functioning primary care system.

First, a good primary care doctor is personally chosen by his or her patients. Doctors who know their patients and have treated them over several years diagnose new problems more accurately and run up fewer costs.

Second, a good primary care doctor is a skilled listener and professional observer able to head off costly problems when they first appear. He or she is an effective counselor, trained in how to get patients to reduce risks in their lives and to manage the on-going health problems that they have.

Third, a good primary care doctor is broadly trained to address the range of problems that constitute 90–95% of the health problems that people of all ages bring to the office. Many academic specialists believe that such a doctor cannot be trained in this era of such vast and complex medical knowledge pertinent to primary care. They always have stories of mistakes by primary care doctors because they end up treating the mistakes rather than all the successes. Their critical stance assumes that if they were doing the primary care, the occasional mistake would not happen. But the fact is that specialists doing primary care make as many or more mistakes. Moreover, the costs and problems of coordination when several specialists combine to cover the spectrum of primary care are greater than if handled by a generalist. Even more to the point is the value of a primary care team with nurse-practitioners and physician assistants with whom many functions can be shared.

Fourth, the good primary care doctor can manage a wide array of services needed by people with disabilities and chronic problems, including home health care and nursing home care. This implies staff skilled in rehabilitation and patient education as part of the primary care team. GP group practices in the UK routinely carry out all these functions. They also draw on an array of other skilled personnel not common in the American system who do community and home nursing.

Fifth, good primary care doctors perform common, uncomplicated procedures such as skin biopsies, sigmoidoscopies, or casting in the office, avoiding referrals and the extra costs entailed.

Sixth, good primary care doctors join specialists in providing care in the hospital and coordinate specialty services. Here, American family physicians are ahead of British GPs, though the recent reforms in the NHS are leading to more coordinated services between GPs and specialists. However, the cardinal rule broken in the American system is that all tests and services should be coordinated through a patient's personal physician, a key to higher quality at lower cost. It requires a single patient file into which all notes, tests, etc. are put, regardless of where the patient is treated and for what.

Small primary care teams provide more choice and flexibility than the huge managed care systems now forming to control America's national health care system. They offer more choice at less cost. Teams as small as four or five generalists together with other clinical staff trained in primary care, community- and home-nursing, patient education, and rehabilitation are all that is needed. Small teams can reflect the ethnic and religious diversity of the nation better than large corporate systems. This is the relevance of the modern British GP group practice to the managed care reform that American leaders seek. If doctors and patients want managed care with a human face, if they want local managed care that reflects the culture and tastes of their community, the broad-spectrum GP group practice demonstrates it can be done.

A number of policy changes are essential in order to develop a sound primary care base for the American health care system. Briefly, they include the following:

- make pay between various specialties more equal

- provide primary care teams with well trained nurses and other providers

- give primary care physicians a distinct role in the delivery system

- increase support for primary care training

- change the curriculum and culture of medical schools

- develop a workforce plan that provides the mix of specialties needed by the population.

Improving Access and Reducing Maldistribution

The US health care system treats the consequences of more inequities, poverty, and social pathology than any other developed country. Exacerbating this problem are serious maldistribution problems in medical services themselves, so that the most disadvantaged and needy are least likely to find accessible services. The increases in physicians per 1,000 population over the past 25 years have not reduced the number of underserved areas; physician maldistribution has only increased. Rural areas have about one-third as many general internists, general pediatricians and obstetricians per 1,000 as metropolitan areas (Bureau of Health Professions). Latino and African-American physicians make up only a fraction of their proportion in the population. The crucial reform to reduce these barriers to access is to cover everyone for needed services so that both doctors and patients are assured of a sound financial base. Further, the nation needs a workforce plan designed to meet the needs of the public, not academic medical departments and directors of residency programs. The National Health Service Corps, which provides scholarships and loan forgiveness to students who commit to practice primary care in underserved urban and rural areas, needs to be revived and supported well. Further, an extensive and early recruitment effort must be mounted to increase the number of applicants from disadvantaged minorities.

Primary Managed Care: a New GP Model

The purpose of this book has been to compare and contrast the primary care systems of two countries. We believe also that there is a great deal we can learn from each other. The recent reforms of general practice in Britain extend regular primary care by giving group practices the budget and capacity to oversee related services. These include home health services, rehabilitative services and physical therapy, drugs, specialty referrals and testing, a set list of elective specialty procedures, and prevention (Grumbach and Fry, 1993; Light and May, 1994). This ambulatory or semi-HMO contract has modest risk limits so that even small groups can qualify. Complementing this fundholding contract are new terms in the general GP contract that pay GPs more for each disadvantaged or deprived patient, and more for meeting targets in preventive services. Moreover, these targets are set for the entire community, not just a doctor's registered practice. The British reforms of primary care are putting them in place nationwide by paying extra for recommended prevention.

This expanded model, for integrating primary care and related services under the clinical management of one's personal physician, might be called Primary Managed Care (PMC). It looks like Figure 8.2. The PMC budget essentially

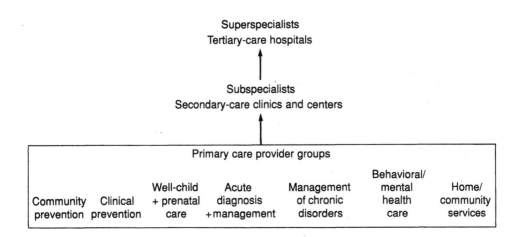

Figure 8.2 A Model of Community-based Primary Managed Care for the 21st Century.

includes everything that most patients with a primary care group practice will normally need. It is not unlike some HMO contracts that give primary care physicians the role for administering the full professional (ie physician) capitation, with independent practitioners, only broader on the chronic-care, home-care side (Cook and Rodnick, 1988).

Primary managed care offers an exciting way to coordinate a wide range of services that are now scattered among different agencies and budgets. It puts broadly trained primary care practitioners in the middle of health care teams focused on health maintenance and medical treatment, with subspecialists and hospitals in reserve when needed.

A rather wide range of diagnostic and treatment services would be delivered by the PMC group. Small groups of physicians (three to 20) would be responsible for all the services contained in the box in Figure 8.2. In the UK, this group receives a negotiated budget from the Regional Health Authority based primarily on the number of patients they care for, weighted by age, a deprivation scale and other factors. The risk would be limited to, let us say, $5,000 per patient per year. It is important to keep the risk meaningful but low, since primary care contracts with high risk can lead to profiteering, underservice, favorable selection, and other distortions. The British also keep risk at a meaningful but modest level by having the population-based capitated payments cover only part of practice costs. Lump-sum allocations cover much of the costs for practice staff and overheads. As previously noted, there are also incentive fees for meeting specific targets in prevention. Lowering the stakes of lump-sum or capitation contracts in these ways not only overcomes the problems of perverse incentives to decrease utilization in capitation contracts by US HMOs (Hillman *et al.*, 1989), but also provides a payment structure for the new paradigm of health care focused on preventing illness and maximizing health gain.

Finally, the British prohibit doctors from pocketing surpluses from their budget; they must go back into the practice. The British view is that medicine is an essential social service, not a business for profit. When some GPs used the reforms to establish for-profit testing and service corporations to which they referred their own patients, Parliament promptly made all such practices illegal. An equally firm stand in the US would return medicine more to a non-profit but adequately paid profession concentrating on the health problems of citizens.

A key step is to encourage primary care physicians to form small groups (or if already in large groups to break into smaller, functional groups) and to have these groups put together primary care teams with nurse practitioners, home visit nurses, and in some cases, social workers and psychologists, to meet the needs of their patients. Bonus payments for team practice should be provided, especially to enhance the features of comprehensiveness of maternal and child health services (Starfield and Simpson, 1993). The beauty of primary managed care is that it is personal, small and local. It is a contractual structure that encourages doctors and other health providers to work as teams. It provides more choice in all areas of the country, particularly in rural areas where large managed care systems either will not form or will constitute a monopoly.

Putting PMC into the US Reforms

These observations suggest that the essence of the reforms should be to provide comprehensive, primary care for every citizen, coordinated by his or her own, personal physician. This central tenet, rather than that of closely regulated competition between large managed care systems run by MBAs (Master of Business Administration), is most likely to control medical costs. Thus, purchasers need to focus on setting up local choices between different PMC teams, while generating competitive bids for more costly and less common secondary and tertiary services for the entire population of a region.

Purchasers should also allocate funds for training health professionals, for evaluating quality and management, for policing services, for clinical research, and for area-wide efforts to reduce risk factors. PMC implies a new way of allocating funds that suits the American values of local control and personal choice. There is complete free choice of one's personal physician by patients and of patients by physicians. It is clinically-managed personal care, not MBA managed corporate care.

At the regional level, PMC contracts for subspecialty services would have to be coordinated so that one neurologist might handle referrals from several PMC groups. Subspecialists could be frustrated if each group had a separate contract, each with different requirements. Less common superspecialty services would be in danger of getting passed over altogether because no one PMC group used them enough to budget for them. This is a logistical problem now being tackled in the second phase of the NHS reforms through area-purchasing consortia (Light, 1994).

PMC and Choice of Physicians

A possible objection to this proposal is that it would reduce 'choice', that is, the ability of patients to choose to go directly to specialists whenever they want. Such choice, however, is medically irresponsible. It means that patients play doctor; they decide what is wrong with them and which subspecialists to see, based on bits of knowledge and inference assembled into a self-diagnosis. The subspecialty mindset maximizes the use of technology and fragmentation and patients' need to decide which opinions and treatments by the subspecialist are right or wrong. Often they know none of these subspecialists well, and sub-specialists do not know them well.

Many times, the subspecialists are members of multi-specialty groups; so the patient finds that he or she is seeing a different person each time and a different subspecialist for each aspect of a complex problem. No one physician has the entire clinical file and neither does the patient. All of them rely on the patient to tell them what action the others are taking as they almost never get together.

Clearly what patients need is a professionally trained advocate and personal protector who knows their history and all their interrelated problems well. It should be the personal physician who advises the patient on the most appropriate specialist to choose, and to refer the patient with a full clinical history and with the expectation of a full report back.

PMC increases choice where it counts, choosing one's personal physician, and makes referral choice a joint effort by patients and their chosen doctors. This is the choice that matters.

The larger goal is to reform American health care as much as possible towards everyone having a personally chosen primary care provider, and to build the health care system around primary managed care. Once a primary care physician has been chosen, annual switching of plans and doctors should not be encouraged because it undermines the key to quality and cost containment. There might even be a switching fee of a few hundred dollars for changing providers, not only because there are in fact real start-up costs to switching, but because there are real losses to holding down health care costs until the new provider gets to know the patient well enough to manage him or her cost-effectively.

More than 30 years ago, Kerr White and his colleagues estimated carefully that, on average, about 750 of every 1,000 people have something they consider an illness or an injury every month (White *et al.*, 1961). Only about 250 of them take their problem to a doctor. Self-care, as we said in Chapter 1, is the most prevalent and most important of the four levels of care. From studies of primary care, however, we know that about half of the 250 come in to see their doctor with self-limiting problems or problems that doctors cannot do much about. Good PMC and community-based efforts should aim at getting that 250 figure down to 150 through patient education, self-management and nurse triage. Parenthetically, when the 250 per 1,000 see specialists rather than generalists, the specialists not only spend more diagnosing and treating them, but they 'find' more things wrong.

Patients should receive comparative data on different practices in clear but objective terms to enhance consumer judgment. Each practice should be required to issue a profile of its services, quality, personnel and prices. Anything beyond that, such as give-aways, jazzy campaigns, and sexy models, runs contrary to true competition, which is to be based on accurate, comparative information about price, quality, and product. All UK general practices must now provide their own printed leaflets stating the services they provide and the staff responsibilities for them.

Downsizing to the Community

Reforms proposed in several bills are based implicitly on regional markets at the level of two to four million people. That level is useful for some macro-level functions but not for dealing with most health care and meeting most health needs. Issues of management and allocation call for a more accessible, less bureaucratic level of decision making.

Chapter 1 pointed out that all systems of health care have four levels of care related to population size and administration. If the US reforms do not make provisions for these levels, they will probably be rediscovered in new guises.

As the US reforms now stand, it will be health insurance companies that will create these vital middle levels at which most critical decisions are made. The problem is that health insurance companies are principally responsible for the adverse selection against people with health problems and for making health coverage precarious for the working and middle classes. It does not bode well for the future to have most health care controlled by companies whose purpose has been to maximize profits for stockholders by discriminating against those who most need medical services.

A more attractive alternative is to structure the health care system so that there are many smaller contracts for many PMC groups. This structure increases choice, flexibility and financial stewardship. Beyond the care these groups provide directly, however, most of these services exist now and will exist at the community or area-wide level. Therefore, funding and coordination of community hospitals, nursing homes, many other service centers and the most frequently used subspecialists should take place at the community level. A good deal of the effective work in reducing risks and in making a community more user-friendly to people with disabilities or chronic problems is also best done locally.

If PMC and community-based services work well, they will significantly lessen the need to ration services, not only by reducing excessive pricing, fraud, duplication, and unnecessary procedures, but also by reducing the frequency of health problems by helping people to cope with them.

Community-based Health Care: the Alternative to Mega-managed Care

Given that most community hospitals, nursing homes and rehabilitation centers already operate at a smaller, more accessible level than regions of two to four million, and given that community-based efforts to reduce health risks, carry out health education, and provide better facilities for people with disabilities also work best, there needs to be a more accessible level of coordination at the community level.

One approach would be community or area-wide health councils overseeing a staff that works to minimize the health and functioning of the local population. This council would deal with managerial and contractual issues, and it would oversee a user-friendly grievance system. It would help focus services on problems that need to be addressed. Community health councils would allow the great diversity of peoples and tastes to be reflected much better than a region that lumps a few million people together into a statistical mass. The councils would also be the critical means by which health status could be improved; for most of the factors that increase morbidity and mortality lie outside medical care. They involve jobs, housing, education, occupational hazards, nutrition and high-risk behavior such as violence, drugs, and alcohol abuse. Once community demands for these services were identified, the councils would be another mechanism to help make the public and other governmental agencies aware of such needs.

Members of community health councils could be elected or appointed, or a mixture of both. Their terms of office should be relatively long, say, four to five years. The people most affected by health services, such as the disabled and chronically ill, should be disproportionately represented. The councils would also have institutional members, especially municipal and county health departments as well as representatives from unions, large employers, the chamber of commerce, welfare departments, the schools, the police, youth services, the churches, and other relevant bodies. The councils should not include providers or managers (nor their families, attorneys or accountants) but utilize them in an advisory capacity. The councils would need a small professional staff and some funds for commissioning expert opinions or studies on difficult issues. A great deal more discussion is needed on the composition and mandates of such community health councils.

These councils, then, would become a critical tool for reducing the incidence of illness. They could also serve a deeper function: to foster dialog and help residents think through their priorities in health care. As Ezekiel Emanuel points out in a seminal book on the ends of human life (Emanuel, 1991), only those affected should decide. Neither clinicians, nor moral philosophers, nor wise men can choose for others how much they value which qualities of their own lives. Do people want, for example, to maximize investments in healthy years and minimize the expenses of prolonging their lives once severely ill? Or does prolonging life take first priority, leaving less for physical medicine and rehabilitation?

As quasi-governmental bodies, community health councils should have some budgetary power. They could become the reconstituted public health system, overseeing those public health programs not taken up in the primary care system and the activities of the regional health alliances. Or they could further have budgetary power for health care service, in which case the flow of funds would look something like the following. Risk-adjusted, capitated budgets would be allocated to regional health alliances from whatever mechanism is set up to collect the funds (taxes, payrolls, or premiums). That body would hold aside and oversee funds for tertiary and other expenses already noted.

Risk-adjusted, capitated budgets for all other care would then be allocated to community health councils. It would then contract with PMC teams, providing the coordination needed for community-based specialty and hospital services. This model of reform has the advantages of:

- increasing choice

- having most health care clinically managed by the physicians responsible for their patients' care

- minimizing large and distant bureaucracies that control health care

- allowing a more flexible structure that can reflect the great diversity among communities

- involving local people in shaping their health care to their values.

In the coming era of functional disabilities experienced by the growing number of elderly, community-wide programs to make the environment less disabling and to meet their needs call for community health councils.

How Much Would Community-based PMC Cost?

Let us consider a budget for 100,000 people. If each primary care physician takes care of 1,500–1,800 enrollees, about 60 primary care doctors per 100,000 population are required. Or, this could be more like 50 doctors and 25 physician extenders (nurse practitioners or physician assistants). If each practice averaged $300,000 to cover each primary care physician plus all the practice overheads (60%), primary care would cost $18 million for a population of 100,000. A further $25 million would be needed for referred subspecialty care. Lastly, $20 million would be required for laboratory work, imaging, home care, physical therapy, ancillary care, podiatry (chiropody), and durable medical equipment not included in the other budgets.

These figures total about $63 million per 100,000 for the care that would be covered by the PMC contract. Additional funds of $5–9 million could be allocated to encourage preventive care, patient education and home-based services. This total comes out to approximately $700 per person per year, before adjusting for patient age or risk factors. Patients would sign up with their personally chosen primary care physician, who would practice in a small or mid-sized group of three to 20 physicians. These groups would be responsible for referring to secondary and tertiary services problems they cannot solve.

Following our argument that it is unhealthy for a patient's personal physician to be put at financial risk while advocating on his or her patient's behalf, the community-based and secondary services outside the PMC contract could be contracted for by community health councils, or by the regional purchasing consortia. The contract with the PMC group might be divided into three parts: one covering direct primary care services, one for secondary and subspecialty services coordinated by the regional alliance or other administrative body, and one for community-based and preventive services, which could be coordinated by the community health councils. Risk as well as rewards could be limited, especially for the second and third parts. Tertiary and uncommon services would be contracted for at the regional or state level.

This arrangement, or something similar, has the great advantage of giving patients and their personal physicians complete choice within a region of the subspecialists, hospitals, and particular centers they decide to use; they would not be locked into the secondary and tertiary services with which a specific, megamanaged care system has contracted. Since the contracting and monitoring of these services would be done at the community-wide or regional level, the patient and doctor are left free to choose as they wish.

The Non-PMC Budget

Assuming 80% of a population is under 65 years of age, they would use about 250 days of hospital care per 1,000 people per year. The 20% of the population, over 65 would use about 1,500 days of care per 1,000. Thus an average US population would use about 500 days of hospital care per 1,000 people per year.

If one capitates hospitals at about \$1,200 per day (in 1993 currency), the cost of hospital care would be roughly \$600,000 per 1,000 enrollees per year \$600 per person. A 200- to 300-bed hospital would be needed if this was an urban or suburban area. Multiple smaller hospitals might be needed in rural areas.

We further estimate that prescription drugs would cost about \$10 million, and dental care, \$12 million for 100,000 people per year. To this should be added \$5 million for health professions' education, \$5 million for outcomes and clinical research, £5 million for public health efforts, \$5 million for skilled nursing facility coverage, \$8 million for administration.

Lastly, we need to add about \$20 million for reserves and contingencies such as transplants, and to cover depreciation and new construction. This subtotal comes to about \$130 million per 100,000 enrollees and would be distributed through contracts and negotiations with the health council.

The total now comes to about \$200 million per 100,000 enrollees per year. Extrapolating for a nation of 270 million people, the national health care budget would be \$540 billion, slightly more than half of what the nation spent in 1993 yet about in line with affluent European nations that provide all needed services, such as Germany, France, and Sweden. Through staged phase-ins over a period of ten years, this kind of downsizing and restructuring is possible.

What Needs to be Done?

First, no health care budget is possible unless everyone contributes according to their household income, and everyone has access to needed and effective health care regardless of their circumstances. It is vital to include everyone before controlling costs, or else costs get controlled by cutting out people and services, as happened during 'cost containment' in the 1980s.

Second, we need the same comprehensive benefits for everyone. If rationing has to take place at some point, it should apply to everyone and not be based on income or health plan.

Third, everyone needs to have a primary care doctor of their personal choosing and primary managed care must be the center of the new American health care system. This is commonly felt to be impossible in the short run because the US has so few primary care physicians. However, as recent analyses (Fielding and Rice, 1993) have shown, the US has nearly as many family physicians, general internists and pediatricians per thousand population as the UK has GPs. The problems lie in their misallocation and underuse in the delivery system.

Without a clearly defined and fundamental role, backed by proper budgeting, even well-trained primary care doctors can only be partially effective in the ways we have described. And without strong supports, they will not work in poor areas. 'The number of doctors willing and eager to practice in the poorest neighborhoods, always inadequate, has dwindled to practically nothing in recent years because of low Medicaid reimbursement rates, the threat of violence and the shifting focus of medical education away from general doctoring and toward specialty training', a recent report on poor areas of New York City concluded (Rosenthal, 1993). A 1990 survey of nine low-income neighborhoods found only 28 properly qualified doctors for 1.7 million people.

Fourth, reforms need to solve the greatest structural problem of American health care: the lack of a clear and central role for primary care physicians in delivering services.

Fifth, the current litigious, malpractice system needs to be replaced with a grievance system which reflects the types of complaints people have and how to rectify them.

Sixth, the training of all health professions needs to be coordinated and changed radically so that schools are oriented to the health needs of communities in the 21st century (Schroeder, 1993). The report by the PEW Health Professions Commission (1991) outlined both the mandate and the changes well. Major organizations now advocate that many more generalists be trained: the American College of Physicians (the professional organization of internists); the American Medical Association (AMA); the Accreditation Council for Graduate Medical Education; the federal government; the National Council of State Legislatures; the National Governors Association; and the Association of American Medical Colleges (who represent medical schools and teaching hospitals).

Changing the mix of physicians (and nurses) to give the US a strong primary care base may be the most difficult part of the plan. Medical training should be tuition-free, but in return society should have the right to have a workforce plan that specifies how many doctors, physician assistants, nurse practitioners, community nurses, physical therapists, and the like it needs. To allow as many students to go into subspecialties as they like not only drives up costs and distorts care, but it amounts to a welfare state for subspecialists; 'You choose what you'd like to do, and we'll pay you $300,000 a year for life.' No other part of the economy works this way. Each young person must balance what he or she is good at with what he or she likes and what society needs. Recruitment must use many more efforts like the National Health Service Corps and the Physician Shortage Area Program in order to recruit students from underserved and rural areas, and have students spend significant time in these areas during their years of training and initial practice.

Finally, primary care needs to be made more attractive. Levelling income inequalities is a key factor. Recent research by William Hsiao, who developed the resource-based relative value scale used to pay doctors in proportion to their costs, efforts, intensity, and training, found that on average the current values underpay primary care doctors for their *practice costs* by $67,000 and overpay specialists by the same amount. On top of that, the overall income of various specialties ranges nine-fold under Medicare and 13-fold under private insurance payments. Even after taking into account the extra costs and two or three years of extra training for subspecialties, they are significantly overpaid. The British have a healthier approach: medical education is free and all subspecialists are paid on the same salary scale so that differentials between primary care and subspecialties are much less than in the US. But making primary care attractive goes beyond take-home pay. The concept of primary managed care would be more attractive because it puts providers at the center of the system, with a budget that enables them to orchestrate most of the care needed by most of the patients. The development of teams makes work more satisfying, and so do opportunities to learn new things.

We can learn from the UK how to make primary care more attractive. For example, the provision of funds for GPs to take continuing medical education courses and to have paid vacations builds morale and knowledge and helps offset the high personal stress of primary care. Generous retirement pensions, indexed to inflation to assure a comfortable life after years of service is another good idea. Another practice that makes primary care more attractive in the UK is its designation as a teaching practice so that students and residents can participate in their practice. This not only makes their life more interesting as hands-on teachers, but they get the prestige and a few extra funds. All these features contribute to having the majority of medical school graduates in the UK go into primary care.

Barbara Starfield has compared primary care systems in ten developed countries. They include the US, the UK, Canada, Germany, and a number of the Scandinavian countries. The criteria for rating primary care included system characteristics such as the type of physician who provides primary care, per cent of physicians who are specialists, income of primary care physicians relative to specialists, and financial barriers to access to primary care. She also rated primary care practice characteristics such as comprehensiveness, coordination of services, continuity of care, family centeredness, and community orientation. In order to rate the 'primary care-ness' of each country, Starfield assigned to each characteristic a score of 0 (for absence of or poor development), 1 (moderate development), or 2 (high level of development). She averaged the scores and produced the results as shown in Table 8.2.

Although we chose the UK and US to study before Starfield's results appeared, we are not surprised that they received the highest and lowest primary care scores, respectively.

There are very strong inverse relationships between a country's per capita expenditures on health and its primary care score, with the UK at one extreme and the US at the other. Starfield has found that the number of hospitalizations, the number of physicians per thousand population, and the physician

Table 8.2 Starfield's primary care score

Country score	Strength of primary care
United Kingdom	1.7
Denmark	1.5
Finland	1.5
Netherlands	1.5
Canada	1.2
Sweden	1.2
Australia	1.1
Belgium	0.8
Germany (West)	0.5
United States	0.2

contacts per capita are unrelated to a country's health care expenditures. What is related is the use of technology and the number of subspecialists.

There is also a general concordance between a country's primary care score, health indicators and people's satisfaction with the health system. Countries with primary care scores above 1 and with high satisfaction scores have better health indices. The US ranks low in all three (as does Germany and Belgium). The Netherlands, Sweden and Canada rank high in all three. The UK, although highly ranked in primary care, has intermediate ranking in satisfaction and a low ranking for health indices. Dr Starfield hypothesizes that this disparity may result from underfunding of hospital care, education and social services in the UK.

Summary

We have stressed that creating a strong foundation of primary care for American health care is a key to holding down costs while providing accessible, high-quality care. This central role of good primary care has led us to propose a different starting point and model for national health care reform, one that can be incorporated into a number of proposals for financial and insurance reform. Primary care should go beyond gatekeeping to being the center of community-based services aimed at improving the health of a defined population. The starting point for health care reform should not be finance or some model of 'managed competition' from the insurance industry. The reforms should start with the nature of services at the individual and local levels.

Primary managed care might be called the *more choice/less cost* approach to reforming not only the American system but a number of other systems where subspecialization and medical technology are driving up costs. There is much about the British system that does not suit the American situation; but the success of their primary care system echoes American successes in such HMOs as Kaiser, Harvard, Group Health of Puget Sound, and Health Insurance Plan of New York. The more choice/less cost alternative to managed competition provides the basis for community-based and regional efforts in public health and health promotion that have been articulated so effectively by the European office of WHO, by the US Surgeon General, and by the Canadian government. It is difficult to imagine surviving the tidal wave of chronicity and health problems approaching the shores of the health care system as the baby boom generations reach old age after 2010 without some form of primary managed care with community health councils to integrate public health, nursing, and general medicine.

References

Aaron HJ and Schwartz WB (1993) Managed competition: little cost containment without budget limits. *Health Affairs.* **12**: 204–15.

Aday L (1993) *At risk in America: the health and health care needs of vulnerable populations in the United States.* Jossey-Bass, San Francisco.

American Academy of Family Physicians (1993) *Facts about family practice.* AAFP, Kansas City.

American Academy of Family Physicians (1992) *Hospital practice characteristics survey.*

American Academy of Family Physicians (1993) *Definitions approved by AAFP Board of Directors,* November.

American Medical Association (1992) *Physician characteristics and distribution in the US.* AMA, Chicago.

Bertakis KD and Robbins JA (1989) Utilization of hospital services. A comparison of internal medicine and family practice. *J Fam Prac.* **28**: 91–6.

Bertakis KD and Robbins JA (1987) Gatekeeping in primary care: a comparison of internal medicine and family practice. *J Fam Prac.* **24**: 305–9.

Blankfield RP, Kelly RB and Alemagno SA *et al.* (1990) Continuity of care in a family practice residency program. Impact on physician satisfaction. *J Fam Prac.* **31**: 69–73.

Blendon RJ and Edwards JN (1991) *System in crisis: the case for health care reform.* Faulkner and Gray, New York.

Bowman MA (1989) The quality of care provided by family physicians. *J Fam Prac.* **28**: 346–55.

Buescher PA, Roth MS and Williams D (1991) An evaluation of the impact of maternity care coordination on Medicaid birth outcomes in North Carolina. *Amer J Public Health.* **81**: 1625–9.

Bureau of Health Professions. *Rural health professions facts: supply and distribution of health professions in rural areas.* Rockville, MD.

Canadian Health Insurance Lessons for US (1991), GAD/HRD 91–90, Washington.

Cherkin DC, Rosenblatt RA and Hart LG *et al.* (1987) The use of medical resources by residency-trained family physicians and general internists: is there a difference? *Medical Care.* **25**: 455–69.

Clinton W (1993) Speech before the joint houses of Congress, 22 September.

Colwill JM (1992) Where have all the primary care applicants gone? *New Eng J Med.* **326**: 387–93.

Consumers Reports (1992) *Health Care Dollars.* New York.

Cook JV and Rodnick JE (1988) Evaluating HMO/IPA contracts for family physicians: one group's experiences. *J Fam Prac.* **26**: 325–31.

Council Graduate Medical Education (COGME) (1992) *Third report.* US Department of Health and Human Resources, Public Health Service.

Cuyler AJ (1991) *Health care and health care finance in Sweden: summary of an international review of the Swedish health care system.* SNS Occasional Paper, Number 33.

Dixon J (1992a) US health care: the access problem. *Br Med J.* **305**: 817–19.

Dixon J (1992b) US health care: the cost problem. *Br Med J.* **305**: 878–80.

Doctors' and dentists' pay review body report (1992) HMSO, London.

Eddy DM (1991) What care is essential? What services are basic? *JAMA.* **265**: 782–6.

Emanuel EJ (1991) *The ends of human life: medical ethics in a liberal policy.* Harvard University Press, Cambridge, Mass.

Enthoven AC (1985) *Reflections on the management of the National Health Service.* Nuffield Provincial Hospitals Trust. Occasional Paper 5, London.

Enthoven AC (1988) *Theory and practice of managed competition in health care finance.* North-Holland, Amsterdam.

Epstein AM *et al.* (1984) A comparison of ambulatory test ordering for hypertensive patients in US and England. *JAMA.* **252**: 1723–6.

Fielding JE and Rice T (1993) Can managed competition solve the problems of market failure? *Health Affairs.* **12**: 216–28.

Franks P and Dickinson JC (1986) Comparisons of family physicians and internists: process and outcome in adult patients at a community hospital. *J Fam Pract.* 24: 152–6.

Franks P, Clancy CM and Natting PA (1992) Sounding board: gatekeeping revisited – protecting patients from over-treatment. *New Eng J Med.* 327: 424–7.

Friedson E (1990) *Profession of medicine.* Dodd, Mead, New York.

Fry J (1969) *Medicine in three societies.* American Elsevier, New York.

Fry J and Orton P (1992) *General practice: the facts.* Radcliffe Medical Press, Oxford.

Fry J (1988) *General practice and primary healthcare, 1940s–1980s.* Nuffield Provincial Hospitals Trust, London.

Fry J and Horder JP (1993) *Primary care in 12 countries: a comparative survey.* Nuffield Provincial Hospitals Trust, London.

Fry J and Sandler G (1993) *Common diseases.* 5th edition. Kluwer, Lancaster.

Gabel LL, Lucas JB and Westbury RC (1993) Why do patients continue to see the same physician? *Family Prac Res J.* 13: 133–47.

Greenfield S, Nelson EC and Zubkoff M *et al.* (1992) Variations in resource utilization among medical specialties and systems of care: results from the medical outcomes study. *JAMA.* 267: 1624–30.

Grumbach K and Fry J (1993) Managing primary care in the United States and in the United Kingdom. *NEJM.* 328: 940–5.

Hainer BL and Lawler FH (1988) Comparison of critical care provided by family physicians and general internists. *JAMA.* 260: 354–8.

Hartley RM *et al.* (1987) Differences in ambulatory test ordering in England and America – role of doctors' beliefs and attitudes. *Am J Med.* 82: 513–17.

Havlicek PL (1990) *Prepaid groups in the US: a survey of practice characteristics.* AMA, Chicago.

Hillman AL, Pauly MV and Kerstein JJ (1989) How do financial incentives affect physicians' clinical decisions and the financial performance of health maintenance organizations? *NEJM.* 321: 86–92.

Hjortdahl P and Laerum E (1992) Continuity of care in general practice: effect on patient satisfaction. *Br Med J.* 304: 1287–90.

Hjortdahl P (1991) Continuity of care: general practitioners' knowledge about, and sense of responsibility toward their patients. *Br Med J.* **303**: 1181–4.

Hjortdahl P (1992) The influence of general practitioners' knowledge about their patients on the clinical decision-making process. *Scan J Primary Health Care.* **10**: 290–4.

Hoffenberg R (1987) *Clinical freedom.* Nuffield Provincial Hospitals Trust, London.

Hsiao WC, Dunn DL and Verrilli DK (1993) Assessing the implementation of physician-payment reform. *New England Journal of Medicine.* **328**: 928–33.

Journal of the American Medical Association, Special Issue (1992) *Graduate medical education: App III.* **268**: 1170–6.

Kohn R and White KL (1976) *Health care: an international study.* Oxford University Press, Oxford.

Kravitz RL, Greenfield S and Rogers W *et al.* (1992) Differences in the mix of patients among medical specialties and systems of care: results from the medical outcomes study. *JAMA.* **267**: 1617–23.

Lee PR, Soffel D and Luft HS (1992) Costs and coverage: pressures towards health care reform. *Western J Med.* **157**: 576–83.

Light DW (1992a) The practice and ethics of risk-rated health insurance. *JAMA.* **267**: 2503–8.

Light DW (1992b) Another look at rationing and technology. *Health Affairs.* **11**: 263.

Light DW (1993) Countervailing power: the changing character of the medical profession in the United States. *In*: Hafferty F and McKinlay J (eds) *The changing character of the medical profession: an international perspective.* Oxford University Press, New York.

Light DW (1994) *Locality-based joint commissioning: challenges and strategies in comparative perspectives.* North West Regional Health Authority, London.

Light DW and May A, eds (1994) *From welfare state to managed markets: the transformation of British medicine.* Faulkner and Gray, Washington.

Linn LS, Yater J and Leake BD *et al.* (1984) Differences in the numbers and costs of tests ordered by internists, family physicians and psychiatrists. *Inquiry.* **21**: 266–75.

MacDowell NM and Black DM (1992) Inpatient resource use: a comparison of family medicine and internal medicine physicians. *J Fam Prac.* **34**: 306–12.

McClure CL *et al.* (1986) Family practice and internal medicine clinical judgement in a university setting. *J Fam Prac.* **22**: 443–8.

Millis JS (1966) The Graduate Education of Physicians. *Report of the Citizens Commission on Graduate Medical Education*. AMA, Chicago.

Moy E and Hogan C (1993) Access to needed follow-up services: variations among different Medicare populations. *Arch Int Med*. **153**: 1815–23.

National Center for Health Statistics (1991) *Health United States, 1990*. US Department Health and Human Resources, Hyattsville, Maryland.

Noren J *et al*. (1980) Ambulatory medical care: a comparison of internists and family general practitioners. *New Eng J Med*. **802**: 11–16.

Office of Health Economics (1995) *Compendium of health statistics*, 9th edition. Office of Health Economics, London.

PEW Health Professions Commission (1991) *Healthy America: practitioners for 2005*. PEW Health Professions Commission, Durham, NC.

PEW Health Professions Commission (1993) *Health Professions Education for the Future: Schools to the Nation*, San Francisco.

Physicians for a National Health Program, Quality of Care Task Force (1993) *Draft report*, 8 November.

Pope GC and Schneider JE (1992) Data watch, trends in physician's incomes. *Health Affairs*, 181–93.

Rabinowitz HK (1993) Recruitment, retention, and follow-up of graduates of a program to increase the number of family physicians in rural and underserved areas. *New England Journal of Medicine*, **328**: 934–9.

Relman AD (1992) Personal communication.

Rice T, Brown ER and Wyn R (1993) Holes in the Jackson Hole approach to health care reform. *JAMA*. **270**: 1257–1362.

Roback G, Randolph L and Seidman B (1990) *Physician characteristics and distribution in the US*. AMA, Chicago.

Rosenblatt *et al*. (1983) The content of ambulatory medical care in the US, an interspecialty comparison. *New Eng J Med*. **309**: 892–7.

Rosenthal E (1993) Shortage of doctors in rural areas is seen as a barrier to health plans. *New York Times*. October 18.

Rubin HR, Gandek B and Robers WH *et al*. (1993) Patients' ratings of outpatient visits in different practice settings. *JAMA*. **270**: 835–40.

Rublee DA (1989) Data watch: medical technologies in Canada, Germany and US. *Health Affairs.* 8(3): 180.

Rublee DA (1992) *International health care systems: a chartbook perspective.* AMA Center for Health Policy Research, Chicago.

Schiff GD and Goldfield NI (1994) Deming meets Braverman: towards a progressive analysis of the continuous quality improvement paradigm. *IJHS.*

Schroeder SA (1993) Training an appropriate mix of physicians to meet the nation's needs. *Acad Med.* **68**: 118–22.

Schroeder SA and Sandy LG (1993) Specialty distribution of US physicians – the invisible driver of health care costs. *New England Journal of Medicine*, **328**: 961–3.

Schwartz WB (1987) The inevitable failure of current cost containment strategies: why they can provide only temporary relief. *JAMA.* **257**: 220–4.

Secretaries of State for Health (1989) *Working for patients.* HMSO, London.

Shieber GJ, Poullier JP and Greenwald LM (1992) US health expenditure performance: an international comparison and data update. *Health Care Financing Review.* **13**: 1–73.

Simpson D, Rich ED and Dalgaard KA *et al.* (1987) The diagnostic process in primary care: a comparison of general internists and family physicians. *Social Science and Medicine.* **25**: 861–5.

Social Trends 23 (1993) HMSO, London.

Sofaer S and Hurwich ML (1993) When medical group and HMO part company: disenrollment decisions in Medicare HMOs. *Medical Care.* **31**: 808–21.

St Peter RF, Newacheck PW and Halfon N (1992) Access to care for poor children: separate and unequal? *JAMA.* **267**: 2760–4.

Starfield B and Simpson L (1993) Primary care as part of US health service reforms. *JAMA.* **269**: 3136–9.

Starfield B (1992) *Primary care: concept, evaluation and policy.* Oxford University Press, New York.

Starr P (1982) *The social transformation of American medicine.* Basic, New York.

Stevens R (1971) *American medicine and the public interest.* Yale University Press, New Haven.

Strauss MJ, Conrad B and Logerfo JP *et al.* (1986) Cost and outcome of care for patients with chronic obstructive lung disease. Analysis by physician specialty. *Medical Care.* **24**: 915–24.

The Economist (1992) *Pocket world in figures.* The Economist Books, London.

White KL, Williams TF and Greenberg BG (1961) The ecology of health care. *NEJM.* **265**: 885–92.

Woolhandler S and Himmelstein DU (1991) The deteriorating administrative efficiency of the US healthcare system. *NEJM.* **324**: 1253–8.

World Health Organization (1978) *Health for All: 2000.* WHO, Geneva.

Index